Mortal Embrace

TRANSLATED BY LINDA COVERDALE

Hill and Wang · New York

A DIVISION OF

FARRAR, STRAUS AND GIROUX

EMMANUEL DREUILHE

MORTAL EMBRACE

LIVING WITH AIDS

Library of Congress Cataloging-in-Publication Data
Dreuilhe, Emmanuel.
Mortal embrace.
Translation of: Corps à corps.
1. Dreuilhe, Emmanuel—Health.   2. AIDS (Disease)—
Patients—United States—Biography.   3. AIDS (Disease)—
Psychological aspects. I. Title.
RC607.A26D7413   1988   362.1'969762'00924   [B]   88-6660

For Joseph Sonnabend
and Donald Kotler

Contents

But we have understood nothing about illness so long as we have not recognized its resemblance to war and to love, its compromises, its feints, its exactions, that strange and unique amalgam produced by the mixture of a temperament and a malady.

—MARGUERITE YOURCENAR
Memoirs of Hadrian

When all the breathers of this world are dead;
   You still shall live—such virtue hath my pen—
Where breath most breathes,
even in the mouths of men.

—SHAKESPEARE
Sonnet 81

Mortal Embrace

PROLOGUE

THE EARTH QUAKED, and the shock wave of AIDS awakened monsters from the depths of our collective imagination, monsters of a species we had long thought extinct. This plague has attracted the inevitable swarm of AIDS researchers, officials, businessmen, and journalists, and they are the ones who have monopolized the media. We people with AIDS, who devote each waking moment to our own survival, have been unable to prevent those loquacious experts from stealing our thunder and robbing us of the only thing we have left: our illness.

Like children whose guardianship is in dispute, or natives whose fate depends on the mysterious workings of distant colonial authorities, we huddle, dazed and terrified, while arguments whistle overhead. Perhaps that is why we tiptoe off, one by one, so as not to be in the way, leaving the grown-ups to continue their discussion among themselves. Healthy people don't need us either: a new trend, another fashionable cause will cast us back into the darkness whence we came.

Like all those with AIDS, I tasted hemlock in my diagnosis. The epidemic had been raging long enough for neighbors, friends, lovers to have vanished discreetly from my life. I was not yet forty, and part of my past had already crumbled under the violent assault of AIDS. Many had been struck down after a few weeks of agony; some, like myself, have been lucky enough (if one can call lucky those prisoners in a concentration camp who weren't gassed right away) to see the passage of several seasons and to have survived some of the opportunistic diseases that prey on us, like so many Furies.

What outsiders say about us is not necessarily false, but I find their words so abstract as to be pointless. Anthropologists of our *tristes tropiques* have accumulated a considerable store of information and conclusions about our genes and our mores, our mode of socialization and our myths, but in so doing, they've lost sight of our humanity.

It's just that they talk about people with AIDS as if we were already lost, already dead. And we all look alike to them too. It's true that in the last stages of our illness all of us seem to have had our portraits done by the same follower of El Greco, who models the features of Rock Hudson and the body of a puny intellectual with an equal ruthlessness. The fallen all weigh the same, all wear the same AIDS mask and the same striped pajamas.

The others see only the dying, and prefer to forget that thousands of us still flutter about at liberty in society, not yet pinned and chloroformed like so many death's-head moths. We've reached the darkest hour, when the scope of this evil is all too evident, when researchers appear to be going around in circles, and when society seems ready to give in to the demons of selfishness and fear. It was in a similar situation, just after the collapse of the European continent, that Churchill sought to inspire hope in a demoralized nation. We're all Londoners under the Blitz, but who will make us believe that our salvation lies in "blood, sweat, and tears"?

And yet these pages, written during a lull between two air raids on a table still quivering from the blasts, could never be the work of anyone else with AIDS. This diary is a singular experience, but I have tried to present, in the manner of David Hockney's photographic montages, a complete series of images of the same sickroom: that mental room which now forms the confined universe of people with AIDS, a room we will leave only to die. All those snapshots with overlapping perspectives offer views that vary according to the day and mood. Here and there a detail might be arbitrarily enlarged, out of proportion to the other elements of the picture, because our perception of our own condition is uneven and discontinuous.

During the months when I was writing this diary of AIDS, I was several different people, and each one speaks in turn in the pages that follow: one moment Fabrizio at Waterloo in *The Charterhouse of Parma*, confused and frightened; the next, Nelson

at Trafalgar—wounded, but lucid. Gathering together these already faded photos has helped distract
me from my morbid contemplation of the seemingly
inescapable lava flow advancing toward me from
Vesuvius. For AIDS is perhaps above all a mental
illness, not so much because the virus may affect our
brains as because it forces upon us such isolation
and anguish that it drives us mad. Since the onset
of my sickness, I have come to understand what a
nervous breakdown can be. The unreality of the
non-AIDS universe of healthy people leads me to
question their common sense and mistrust my own
senses. Like the homeless derelicts of New York
City, talking to themselves as they push along their
nauseating shopping carts, we inspire a mixture of
disgust and pity, and like them, we know that what
surrounds us is not—or at least ought not to be—
reality.

And so I wasn't quite in my right mind when I
began to compose these fragments of a warrior's
discourse addressed to the only protagonist who
understands me, to the Sphinx who has set me to
solve the ultimate riddle of my existence, to my last
love: AIDS.

My personal war began two years ago when I was
mobilized by AIDS. All the pleasures of peacetime
and my carefree life were suddenly banished, as if
an orchestra had stopped playing to let the theater
manager announce that war had just been declared,

that Pearl Harbor had been bombed. Since then I
have devoted myself exclusively to the war effort,
because the futility of civilian life (my thirty-six years
of good health) is absurd when survival itself has
become the main imperative. Proust likened Germany and France to two organisms locked in conflict, and he identified with France in his stormy
relationship with the treacherous Albertine, whose
scheming he compared to German military strategy.
AIDS is my Albertine, a frightful, intimate enemy,
like a demon or familiar spirit. Since the moment
we met, I've been obliged to keep my decks cleared
for action (no more fooling around with sailors),
and I've invested everything in war bonds for our
Defense Department: hospitals and medical specialists. I might even hoist defiant flags over the
already invaded organs of my body, which has become a battlefield like Paris in 1871, torn between
the opposing forces of the Commune and the Prussians. On this same corporal survey map, I could
also indicate the organs once believed lost to the
enemy but retaken after bitter fighting, backed up
by an artillery barrage of antiviral and sulfa drugs:
chemical weapons in that trench warfare which has
kept me pinned down for almost two years now.
Soon eight seasons will have come and gone, without a sign of peace or victory on the horizon. I'm
already a war casualty, disfigured by my wounds,
but I must go on fighting, disabled as I am. What

other struggle is so fierce that it rages even inside hospitals?

The enemy is not so much the HIV virus itself—supposing that it is the only cause of AIDS—as it is the unshakable conviction of the media, public opinion, my father, all my friends and allies—when they're being honest with themselves—a conviction that a part of me shares: that AIDS, as the press keeps repeating, "is an illness that is always rapidly fatal and for which there is no cure." I believe in myself, just as the besieged Communards loved France, and in a sense it isn't the Prussians that are my enemies, but the defeatist and overly rational troops of the Versailles government. Like them, men and women with AIDS are tempted to surrender just to get it all over with as fast as possible, even at the risk of losing their self-respect. If I start to be "reasonable," I'm finished, because the statistics leave no room for hope. I must fight one against ten, like Roland battling the Saracens, and die like a valiant knight, hypodermic in hand.

We have grown up in our bodies, they are our native lands, and although we know their short-comings by heart, we have a natural affection for them, warts and all. My country has occasionally disappointed me, but like a Resistance fighter, I'll stop at nothing when it comes to throwing off the foreign viral yoke. The main thing is to adopt a guerrilla attitude and reverse our roles. To declare that imposters have taken over my body, that the virus has illegally usurped authority, and that I must set out to recover my morale and all biological ground lost so far. I'm in my own home, this is my body, and it's up to AIDS to get out. Illness has given each of my organs a hitherto unsuspected importance. When France was invaded on her eastern border, the names of insignificant towns like Verdun, which meant nothing to French citizens before the war, suddenly took on an overwhelming symbolic value. The Marne was no longer that innocuous river where one went to try a little fishing or stroll about with the family, but became instead a crucial line of defense against the enemy. In the same way, I now find that my eyes, my bowels have acquired a new and vital importance since coming under attack. Illness is a voyage of discovery through the body that makes you marvel at how harmoniously it functioned in the good old days, before the virus had begun its withering assault. Now the corpses of our two armies drift down through my intestines, which threaten to run as red with blood as the Moskva during the retreat from Russia. This illness has led me to adopt Kennedy's patriotic slogan as my own: I must ask no longer what my body can do for me, but what I can do for my body, whose each and every cell is precious to me. In my

mythology, my eyes, harassed by the cytomegalovirus, might well be my Alsace and Lorraine, prov-
inces almost lost to the enemy.

Even though I've decided that I will not die and
that I'll expose, perhaps even confound, the proph-
ets of doom, I'm tempted to see in my illness (which
could have been different: cancer, multiple sclerosis)
a kind of epilogue, a time to take stock of my life.
Held at bay by the enemy, with my back to the
sickroom wall, I can take a breather, and I find that
I enjoy an exceptional lucidity, at least for the time
being. As I sift through the rubble of my shattered
life, I find here a childhood memory of an outing
on the Saigon River, there a disappointed youthful
dream, elsewhere one of Kristine's mischievous
smiles, or an expression of abandon on Oliver's face.
Then, farther on, I rediscover the mysterious axis of
the avenues through Angkor Wat, which my family
used to visit during Easter vacation. Archaeologist
of my own past, I try to discern what has been the
guiding principle of my life, my *voie royale*, the
road—sometimes high, sometimes low—that has
led me to prolong an exile already chosen by my
parents and to live far from the land whose culture
has nourished me. France, the country I thought I
had left behind, from which I had happily made my
escape, has returned in force, like a mother whom
I might have long kept coolly at a distance and who
would have flown at once to my bedside at the news

of my illness. This culture and my body, which I used so ungratefully, are the two pillars still standing to which I cling, holding on with all my rage to live in an effort to escape being swept away by the vast mudslide of AIDS.

For a long time, I was a deserter. Now where could I go, I who have been around the globe several times? My wandering stops here, and my contradictions blow up in my face. The pacifist who managed to avoid the draft now stands at attention, humming martial tunes. The citizen of the world turns out to have unsuspected Albigensian roots. The Proustian porch of the church of St.-André-des-Champs has taken me to its heart, whereas the Empire State Building can be of no help. I would never have been able to write this book in English, because an adopted language can still betray you. Raised amid the chorus of exotic tongues of our former colonial empire, I knew, from the moment of my infant stammerings, that my first and last hope would lie in the language of my family, the language of France.

PANORAMA
IN TROMPE L'OEIL

ILLNESS IS FORESEEABLE only in hindsight.
It begins with simple skirmishes at the frontier gar-
risons—a bad case of flu, a lingering bronchitis—
but one ignores the warnings of fate and the press,
one goes on living as before, squandering strength
and energy on peacetime pursuits: physical exercise,
leisure activities, seduction (like officers at a military
post who keep chasing skirts as they await the Tartar
hordes—which do arrive, in the end, and along the
expected route across the steppe). No one had realized that behind these minor border incidents, the
ineffectual antibiotics, the intermittent fever, lies the
steely determination of German aggression. I was
somewhat like the Popular Front government,
caught up in the pleasures of pacifism, and then
suddenly the ultimatum is delivered: suppressor T
lymphocytes are massed threateningly on the border, while lavish social spending has depleted our
reserves of T4 + lymphocytes, the immune cells of
our Maginot Line. In my case, the illusion of in-
vulnerability included my conviction that the Americans were more fragile than I, a Frenchman who
had survived the colonies' worst tropical illnesses. I

thought that this shield of immunity would suffice to protect me from the arrows of AIDS. A bit like France in 1939, resting on her laurels from World War I. After a few artillery exchanges, all hell breaks loose: it becomes clear that Hitler is backed up by a powerful war machine, and now panic sets in.

The gross inequality of the opposing forces and the extent of the sacrifices that lie ahead are not immediately apparent. Of course, the general public has been aware since 1981 of the first inroads made by AIDS, thanks to the alert sounded by the press, but the battlefront was still quite distant then, and its victims probably none too clever. They were raw recruits, whereas we're now the Old Guard, seasoned veterans of the Russian campaign. The media have even sensationalized the situation, if that's at all possible, and every week their communiqués announce the death toll, just as they did during the Vietnam War. So many dead, so many wounded, state by state, city by city, country by country. The enemy gives no quarter: the wounded are finished off with bayonets. Gradually, it's true, we learn to recognize the enemy's tactics, if not its strategy, and we gain a better idea of its strong and weak points (yes, there are weak points). Phalanxes spring up under the banner of their battalions: the Sonnabend Battalion, the Kotler Brigade—named after my doctors, whose AIDS patients form a devoted corps under their command. I see them marching in close order; many are cut down, but the survivors continue to advance. They have no choice, even though the ground beneath their feet is often mined. Some, like Oliver, still healthy and seemingly far from the front, step on a mine and are suddenly gone, while others die piecemeal, losing first an ear, then an arm or leg, perhaps a lung, and still they press on regardless, their eyes filmy from the ravages of CMV, half blind, half mad, hallucinating from the effects of medicines as much as from the enemy's bacteriological weapons.

For quite some time, I've been beginning my letters to friends with "News from the Front." A strange army indeed, in which merit is conferred only by length of service, even though chance plays an admittedly important role here. And another thing: instead of a general mobilization, we draw lots, like they did under the Ancien Régime, except that now the rich can't hire paupers to replace them on the battlefield. Still, combat conditions are more or less comfortable, depending on one's social rank, although cannonballs sometimes drop in on headquarters (I've known doctors who've died of AIDS). I tend to judge my fellow patients according to martial criteria, especially since watching Oliver die after only three months of combat. Blitzkrieg. Oliver was a bit like Bara, that brave little soldier of republican legend who kept his mouth shut under royalist torture, without ever really understanding what the grown-ups were fighting about. In the movies, we admire the strong, silent types, men whose faces betray excruciating pain through a slight clenching of the jaw muscles. Oliver was killed in action; he died without shedding a tear, holding his mother's hand. From here into eternity. I've also known the camaraderie of brothers-in-arms at the hospital of La Salpêtrière in Paris, where the fact of belonging to a special team of marines engaged in a daring antiviral counterattack (Pasteur Institute code number HPA23), with its risks of toxic side effects, made us all commandos trying out the latest in experimental weaponry deep behind enemy lines. Like all recruits everywhere, we complain about the macrobiotic grub while swigging from a communal flask of lecithin.

One of the virtues most highly prized in an AIDS patient is a sense of humor, an attitude that is always emphasized in a war film, where we're supposed to admire the guys who crack jokes with the nurse and banter sardonically with the doctor while having their legs amputated. A last revenge against fate: warding off terror by whistling in the dark, like Victor Hugo's Gavroche singing "Blame it on Voltaire!" while under fire in *Les Misérables*. In both cases, humor is an unconscious process that defuses fear, dares to speak of the unspeakable, and represents, despite its morbid appearance, an affirmation of life. AIDS patients sometimes embarrass medical personnel and others around them with the frank coarseness of certain gruesome or scatological jokes, the kind soldiers like best. It's just that the presence of danger breaks down many barriers. Refined speech is out of place when the sheets are filthy and your veins are collapsing. Of course, we worry about the health and safety of our neighbors, even as we hope, being only human, that the fatal bullet will cut down someone else, whose eyes we'll close respectfully before we take up our weapons to set out once more, tears still streaming down our wasted cheeks.

For the moment, the enemy has the upper hand, but the Resistance is getting organized; we must play for time, holding on until the great day when the Americans land in Normandy (the trick is to last that long, and it's not easy, as Anne Frank found out). Our bodies are occupied territories, and only fierce resolution keeps us from losing all hope. Is it 1941 or 1943? How can we tell, when they inform us that 150,000 will die in five years, and at the same time announce that a miracle cure will be along within the next three? It's not a good idea to give definite deadlines to soldiers in the field; they might assign limits to their endurance and then become discouraged when the allotted time passes without bringing victory any closer. In 1914, most of the combatants believed the war would be won or lost in a few months, or even weeks.

It really is World War III: according to the World Health Organization, 165 countries are now at war with this new virus, which didn't officially exist until it claimed its first victims, but which has introduced a new kind of war and turned the international situation upside down by realigning all our *cordons sanitaires*. Our Russian front of forty-five years ago, distant but crucial, is now in Zaire, the Philippines, or Brazil, all at grips with a common enemy and struggling to defend themselves according to their varying degrees of development and organization. The press keeps us informed of the advances and retreats of various battlefronts and usually tends to play up atrocities committed by the enemy, which goads us on to further action but also somewhat undermines our morale.

Eisenhower, Montgomery, and de Gaulle did not get along well together—not to mention Stalin. The allied anti-AIDS headquarters is also divided against itself: under the leadership of Montagnier, the French at the Pasteur Institute have strongly criticized (up until their recent armistice) Gallo and his American team, who shamelessly claimed credit for victories won by their official allies. In such situations, the Good Soldier Schweik had better ignore the pitiful shenanigans of those who are supposed to be saving his neck. I'm sorry now that I ever read a magazine article about the internal conflicts within the Federal Centers for Disease Control in Atlanta, the American Los Alamos for AIDS; that's how I learned after the fact of the indifference some of my field marshals displayed toward the human needs of their patients. It was chilling to read that these researchers, our only official hope, are often completely obsessed by their personal or professional rivalries, or by the lucrative potential of their work. The article mentioned a researcher who would destroy the test tubes of one of his competitors every night to delay publication of the results of his experiments. He preferred to impede the overall progress of research rather than allow a rival to make a discovery that might bring him great public acclaim. And all these specialists fight bitterly over the available funds and personnel, which are always inadequate, thereby losing sight of the very purpose of their collective effort. I'm reminded of the egotism of the senior officers in *Paths of Glory*, or the tragic quarrels among the Allies that led to a withdrawal in the Ardennes during the winter of 1944–45, thus delaying the Nazi defeat by precious weeks.

When will another Oppenheimer discover the fearsome weapon that will resolve this internal dissension and sweep the virus from the face of the earth? How long must we wait for our Hiroshima, the drastic remedy they keep promising us, which will inevitably shower us with its own toxic fallout?

Our confidence in technology is rudely shaken when we find ourselves powerless to prevent an epidemic such as AIDS from ravaging the entire world. Our generation thought, in its innocence, that all diseases were curable, just as we thought until recently that there would be no more conventional wars, only nuclear conflicts, technological wars launched by push button and waged for a mere few hours between experts. We thought we had finished with those medieval epidemics that once wiped whole cities off the map (like San Francisco, which has lost more inhabitants to AIDS than to all the wars waged during the city's history). Just when we had counted on being able to leave everything to the professionals and their technological arsenals, we're stunned to discover that we must fight with cold steel, hand to hand as in the old days, with only our own courage and personal resources to fall back on in the end. It's a duel with the Angel of Death, out on the narrow gangplank of the human immune system, not an exchange of long-range missiles. The terror of AIDS lies in the collapse of our faith in technology.

If I was led, unconsciously at first, to compare this epidemic to a war, it's because the participants are mostly men—at least in the developed countries. True, more and more women and children are being afflicted with AIDS, but to me they seem much like civilians massacred by the enemy before they could be evacuated to safety. Women are often presented as the victims of men who have infected them, either

bisexuals or IV drug users. And so it is the mas-
culine—if not the virile—sex that predominates in
the community of researchers and politicians, activ-
ists and priests that has sprung up around the army
of AIDS patients, also largely composed of men.
Women have essentially served as mourners (*Stabat
Mater*), allowed at last into the private life of the
sick person, who had carefully kept them at a distance before he fell ill. Women are afraid of the
enemy because they cannot confront it head-on, and
they fall prey to disturbing rumors, filtering back
from the battlefield, of women's combat units
sighted among those conscripted by AIDS. The het-
erosexualization of the conflict actually signifies its
feminization. Women would like to remain neutral,
like Sweden or Switzerland: wishing us the best of
luck but, with a few exceptions, avoiding all contact
with whatever's going on among all those men.

There are also black regiments in the war against
AIDS, just as there were in the American Army in
the days before integration. These men and women,
who comprise one half of the New York contingent,
are usually heterosexual drug addicts who used contaminated needles. They're fighting on the same side
as I am, but once again, there's a deep division between blacks and whites. There are white drug addicts suffering from AIDS, of course, but I've
noticed while in the hospital that many AIDS patients are black heterosexuals. The soldiers in this

Foreign Legion are often considered to be the dregs of society; they're not from the same respectable milieu as the homosexual lawyers, teachers, students, merchants, and white-collar workers. This "Harlem brigade," without education or employment, seems to have enlisted in the epidemic for lack of career perspectives. Their AIDS is a manifestation of the despair that permeates their lives. There is little contact between these two armies, which too often ignore or even despise each other. Lacking both social and financial resources, the legions of drug addicts are even worse off than the homosexuals. Penniless objects of public charity, these junkies often display an instinctive distrust of the authorities and medical institutions that have traditionally tried to reform them, and they don't even know where to look for help. They're burnt-out cases to begin with, hopeless and suicidal, so that AIDS arrives as the final blow: once more, life has betrayed them.

Laboring under this double disadvantage, the African contingent loses a greater proportion of victims than the army of white homosexuals, and the black soldiers succumb quicker, too, since their drug-ravaged bodies are in much worse shape than those of the well-fed and health-conscious homosexuals. A heterosexual doctor once told me that he felt more closely involved with those of his AIDS patients who came "from a good background" (meaning the white homosexuals) than with those

who were addicts. Doctors sometimes despair of
making any progress with these ragtag troops who
manage to stay on drugs even in the hospital.
They're expendable, and they know it. When decid-
ing who will benefit first from the latest addition to
their medical arsenal, headquarters will give priority
to the more disciplined patients instead of the un-
derprivileged addicts. A disproportionate number
of blacks were also casualties in Vietnam; then as
now, however, in Vietnam as with AIDS, the media
tended to focus on the suffering that was most pre-
sentable to American society, meaning the suffering
of middle-class whites. This predilection for "good"
AIDS victims is doubtless well intentioned, meant
to influence popular opinion by publicizing the
more acceptable elements of the AIDS tragedy so
that society can identify, at least in part, with their
fate. The fact remains that the blacks wind up as
simple cannon fodder, ingloriously dumped into a
common grave. Still, a general mobilization does
bring different social classes together in the barracks,
and mixes varied "types" of homosexuals in doctors'
waiting rooms. There we make new friends and
sometimes find new lovers, a group as disparate as
the French prisoners of war in *Grand Illusion*: the
actor and the engineer, the aristocrat and the peasant, all united in their opposition to the common
foe. I'm quick to feel a certain solidarity with those
on the same firing line as I, even though it may

sometimes be a bit forced. We set off for the front shoulder to shoulder, some weeping and clutching hysterically at their neighbors, others charging with drawn swords, determined to command respect and leave behind an untarnished image of themselves. During our bivouac conversations in moments of calm, as we talk about our families at home, our past lives, our hopes for the future, now and again we compare medicines and swap stories about various drug treatments. Will the general boldly attack the enemy or beat a prudent retreat? Brothers-in-arms who curse their common lot, after all, each one of us dreams of leaving the platoon far behind, of being the sole survivor of a battalion cruelly devastated by the winter onslaught of pneumonia. That's why we stare so gravely at those mysterious X rays of our lungs, aerial views of our situation brought to us by the medical intelligence service.

Finally, this society of men does without sex, at least in theory, like an army marooned on the front line without camp followers. An army is not supposed to make love. In 1917 the American authorities were shocked to discover that the French Army provided brothels for its soldiers in the combat zone. Is that when the first prophylactics were distributed? Now we're all wearing the mental chastity belt of AIDS.

THE TROJAN HORSE

THE PARADOX, in my case, is that the disease has introduced an element of excitement and suspense into a life threatened by the mediocrity and materialistic pleasures of New York. In short, mobilized by the virus, I find I'm a different man. Danger is intoxicating. I can prove and even flaunt my gallantry, my courage, with an ostentation never afforded to me in times of peace.

There are some who discover a vocation for soldiering on the battlefield itself and who flourish under appalling conditions. Struggling to survive, I've learned how precious life is to me, all life, especially my own. It's our native land, after all. At the end of a medically satisfactory day, I often feel euphoric. I've made it through yet another battle, although it won't be the last one in my illness, not by a long shot. It's thrilling to experience survival as a state of grace, to be an elementary force in action, a force as devoid of consciousness as the virus itself. Certain AIDS patients seek to achieve this particular state through yoga and meditation, like samurai before a battle, or the Christian knights, who fasted and prayed before going out to meet the enemy. I read in Jung that the experience of combat has sometimes cured obsessional neuroses, and that is perhaps what has happened in my case, but for each neurotic cured—and at what cost—how many new ones are created? If a miracle cure were found, I would certainly fall into the same depression that often overwhelms war heroes like the fighter pilots of the RAF, who were faced with returning to a routine civilian life devoid of glamour and excitement.

Rather than think about post-AIDS problems, though, I'd do better to admit that I've lost ground in the last six months: the collapse of Oliver, my ally on the left flank, has opened up a new front, both materially and psychologically. The enemy has dropped defeatist propaganda leaflets well behind my defenses: "He surrendered, so why don't you?" I'm trying to bring this pocket of despair under control with V-2 missile bombardments of AZT, an antiviral drug. The loss of my companion, whose death on the battlefield I witnessed in our own home, has filled me with a thirst for revenge, a profound hatred for the virus that killed him and for the society that looked on his struggle with indifference, even a touch of revulsion. His death has made me a diehard Resistance fighter against AIDS. Since I've decided that any opposition, any pressure brought to bear on me—even in a friendly way—risks hampering the general momentum of my personal war effort, I have become ruthless with people who annoy me, even with the best intentions, oblig-

ing me to be polite and civilized like those still on
the home front, who are unaware of the dangers I
face. What I never dared, back when I was healthy,
comes easily to me now, without compunction.
Anyone not with me is against me, which explains
my growing choosiness in my relationships with
people; at the slightest sign of stress, I break it off.
Bothersome people almost play into the hands of
my enemy, like a kind of fifth column, without re-
alizing how serious the situation is. Because once
the disease has broken out, the world is no longer
the same. After Sarajevo, our world crumbled, and
another one took its place; my life has been changed
in the same way, changed forever, even if I do "come
back" someday.

I've heard that for cancer, especially with children,
they've been using visualization techniques that encourage the patients to imagine scenes depicting
their fight against the illness, their own struggle to
get well. As for me, I've been working on my am-
ateur photo album for three years now: some of the
pictures are bad for my morale, whereas others are
like precious amulets. At first, for example, I made
the mistake of thinking we were all like prisoners of
war who weren't even trying to escape because the
foe seemed so invincible. With luck, the most we
could hope for was keeping in touch with our far-
off comrades hooked up to hospital intravenous
tubes. I've come to understand since then that even

though the enemy seems to have temporarily im-
mobilized us, we must try to organize our great
escape, although it may seem like a lost cause. For
our own safety, we mustn't wait any longer for others to come and rescue us or be content with trying
to survive until they get here. The war isn't over,
and passivity will only sap our will to live. True, any
escape attempt requires very serious preparation,
like Edmond Dantès plotting his way out of the
Château d'If in *The Count of Monte Cristo*, but we
need myths like that, to sustain us and give meaning
to an otherwise futile battle.

In my moments of panic, I see AIDS as a tank
pulverizing everything in its path, rolling over all
the barricades erected by medicine as if they were
made of straw, as indifferent to cries for mercy as it
is to the snapping of limbs crushed by its passage.
This fleeting apparition hurts me more than all the
media hysteria.

Wars have always disturbed the mental balance of
combatants who showed no signs of neurosis in
civilian life. The shock of this disease has led me,
and many others with AIDS who can afford the
fees, to consult a psychoanalyst. It was during my
therapy that all these martial metaphors came to me,
and I began to think along the lines of a strategist
or guerrilla fighter. I told my therapist that the cruel-
est thing about my situation was the feeling that I
was fighting alone, while the rest of the world went

on living as if nothing had changed. My comparisons helped me both to express my will to live and to vent my bitterness.

If I were to go now to the gay beach on Fire Island or a nightclub like The Saint in New York, I'd feel like a soldier briefly back on leave from a hellish battlefront who sees all the shirkers, the "queers" who haven't been called up yet, hanging out and partying in a decadent, end-of-the-world atmosphere. I'd feel resentment and contempt, fed by an empty feeling of moral superiority, thinking of those who are already dead and perhaps already forgotten, with just a quick shovelful of earth tossed over their ashes (the funeral homes here refuse to embalm the remains of AIDS victims and insist on cremating them instead). Life goes on, of course, and the sensual appetites of those whose sexual practices still put them at risk are heightened by the very danger itself. I know it's irrational of me to think this, but I unconsciously attribute the good fortune of these draft dodgers to some kind of dark dealings with the devil: they must have connections with someone high up in headquarters. There's no room for tolerance in war, or justice. *Dieu est mon droit* and *Emmanuel über Alles*. The war is being waged on my own territory, just as it was for France in 1914. It's true that the virus has no homeland, unless it might be nothingness—coming suddenly out of nowhere as it did. So I try to push my AIDS back

across the Rhine into harmlessness, into that latent
state where it vegetated in me for years, according
to my doctor.

To describe my pre-AIDS situation, I used to
choose a metaphor quite often used by healthy carriers: I was a walking time bomb. We were a weapon
directed against ourselves but also against society,
trapped as we were in a surrealistic war in which
the soldier is the battlefield, the gun, the enemy, and
the innocent victim, all at once. This walking time
bomb is as dangerous as a loose cannon used to be
on a sailing vessel, careening around the deck and
blindly mowing down everyone in its path.

Whenever I'm tempted by those pleasures now
prohibited by the explosive charge I carry inside me,
I tell myself that the military have seized control of
my inner sanctum. The rebels have no more private
life, because the slightest weakness might betray
them. No ifs, ands, or buts: all civil liberties are
suspended, and all leaves are canceled. Curfew has
been declared: I must be in bed every evening before
midnight. I'm on special rations because even eating
has ceased being a pleasure and become instead a
military exercise aimed at quelling my attacks of
diarrhea—which are like bombardments raining
down on grain-storage silos or fuel tanks. These vital
strategic resources must be held safely in reserve,
these pounds of my flesh I try desperately to keep
from melting away. The disease has cut the Gordian

knots of my former life by imposing a very simple mode of existence upon me. I've been forced into close contact with nature, the elements, primitive forces, and the structure of my own body. Isn't that why recruits must be naked for their physicals, as naked as patients waiting to receive their hospital gowns? For me, AIDS has been a barbarian invasion, a domination of the physical over the moral, a forcible subjection of my sensibilities. A body wracked with pain becomes as barbarous as a country torn apart by war. I admit that I'm a little fascinated by this violence, like Genet admiring the German soldiers in the Paris Métro.

Proust wrote in *The Past Recaptured* that Parisian high society during the Great War was more glittering than ever; fashionable ladies seized every opportunity to give splendid parties ingeniously organized as charity affairs in honor of those they called "our valiant boys at the front." Similarly, fund-raisers for AIDS held on Fire Island and in discos are getting more and more glamorous. People are more generous, it's true, when they're having a good time. Some cruising even goes on at these charity evenings, and New York has an ample supply of patron ladies from the in crowd who never miss a party, AIDS groupies waving aloft the shrouds of our heroic dead. On Broadway you can also see the AIDS equivalent of *Platoon*, "special interest" plays and films that present—oh so delicately—a somewhat distorted picture of this ghastly epidemic. The audience lines up for tickets with a clear conscience, like Proust's Madame Verdurin dunking a brioche in her cocoa while devouring the newspaper account of the sinking of the *Lusitania*.

As for me, when I wish to feel less isolated and lonely, I prefer to think of the humble and heroic behavior of mothers like Julia, who even offered to take care of me after Oliver's death. Following the example of the Larivières in Proust—that simple French couple who left their quiet retirement to help their newly widowed daughter-in-law run her refreshment stand during the war—she would have handed me the bedpan the way the Larivières washed dishes, with a discreet unselfishness. The mothers of POWs in Vietnam wore badges. In California, in the plastics factory where I worked as a stock boy in the summer of 1972, I saw women who wore this badge on their work uniforms. In 1917, in the small towns of America, each family that had sent a soldier off to France proudly displayed a photograph of their hero in a front window for all to see. The mothers of AIDS patients, however, try to conceal from their friends and neighbors the fact that their sons are ill, because revealing the illness would mean admitting that their children belong to one of the high-risk groups stigmatized by society and risking being shunned for having chosen to stay in contact with them, which is what happened to the mother of a friend of mine. Often they even try, as Julia did, to keep the cause of death secret, and they ask the doctors to write down some other illness on their sons' death certificates. Like the Mothers of the Plaza de Mayo in Argentina, some women get together and organize demonstrations to protest the disappearance of their children while society looks the other way, cowed by fear. Such victims ask for it too. So Oliver didn't officially die on the battlefield of AIDS: he's a *desaparecido*, treacherously struck down by the death squads. Most of the martyrs in this war never receive a Purple Heart or any other military honors, and they can't even count on a posthumous rehabilitation. No cheering crowd salutes the departing heroes with last gifts of homemade delicacies and provisions for the road, as civilians did during the American Civil War. There's no general enthusiasm for this shameful campaign.

The difference—supposing that it is one, after all—between AIDS and a war is that we feel as though we're dying for no reason, whereas soldiers are supposed to have a cause worth dying for. Most combatants fight to defend themselves and their homelands, which amounts to the same thing. To have a fighting chance at victory, a soldier must feel he has right on his side. Anyone who feels guilty about having AIDS is like the French pacifists sent to Algeria, or the American blacks who didn't believe in the Vietnam War: they could only fight halfheartedly, and we know what happened as a result. In a way, it's best to be like Ho Chi Minh, to view the enemy as evil incarnate; or to fight as savagely as kamikazes, the way some AIDS victims do; or again—as in my case—to soldier on with the clear conscience of the Americans in World War II. A victory for my democracy.

How can one win without being armed with the faith and fighting spirit of the Mujahedin or the Vietcong? How can homosexuals and drug addicts feel patriotically inspired in their private war when they don't even like themselves, or may actually hate themselves because of a self-image that reflects society's contempt for them? If the opinion of others finally convinces you that you are morally or physically deficient, how can you believe in yourself or in the importance of your own survival? The first reflex of groups stigmatized by society, such as the Jews, is to feel beaten—almost guilty—right from the start, and so they climb meekly into the Nazis' boxcars. In the same way, many AIDS patients give up without a fight, as if they felt they were somehow getting only what they deserved. Yesterday it was the Jews, today it's the people with AIDS: the authorities have acted with the same casual reluctance. I'm appalled by the indifference, often tinged with contempt, of many heterosexuals who remind me of the German petty bourgeoisie, vaguely anti-Semitic, who watched their Jewish neighbors being taken away and refused to get involved, perhaps out of fear but also because deep down they were tempted to see a certain justice in the Nazis' actions. Before AIDS, popular opinion held that homosexuals were enjoying more than their share of the good life, just as Nazi propaganda portrayed the German and Austrian Jews as being too rich and successful.

In *Shoah*, Claude Lanzmann's film about the Holocaust, we see Polish peasants who still complain, even today, that the Jews in their village, gassed to death forty years before, had exploited them and had never worked with their hands. They also attributed the beauty of Jewish women to the time and money they could afford to spend on pampering themselves, unlike the Polish women, whose jealousy is still strikingly apparent. Some heterosexuals resent the fact that homosexuals don't have to take on the same responsibilities as they do (we've never had to take a child to the dentist on a cold and rainy day, or cut back on our "self-indulgent" lifestyles to support an entire family). The hoariest cliché, even within liberal circles, had pre-AIDS gays thinking of nothing but dancing and making love, squandering their money on silly trifles. Homosexual grasshoppers. The compassion felt by many heterosexuals, in the United States and elsewhere, is mitigated by a vague and unhealthy satisfaction rooted in unacknowledged envy.

The healthy population is thus just as terrified of

coming in contact with AIDS victims as the non-Jews of occupied Europe were of associating with Jews, and perhaps sharing their fate. People with AIDS must fight alone, often severely hampered by the unconscious ambivalence they feel toward their own natures. There are many more gay homophobes than there are Jewish anti-Semites, which explains why so many of them give up so quickly. Homosexual or drug-addicted AIDS patients are much more likely than those suffering from cancer or other illnesses to believe their former way of life makes them responsible for their own plight, because most of them have been unable to break free from the restrictive bonds of a traditional mainstream education and they still see their own behavior as somewhat immoral. Imagine a Jewish child in a Catholic school where the teachers would constantly blame his ancestors for crucifying Christ: if the child fell ill and were nursed by these devout Catholics, how could he possibly feel that his life was worth living! That's what happens to homosexuals brought up in a heterosexual society that strongly condemns their lifestyle. They are at fault in their very essence. If nature declares war on them, they have very few allies, and must be prepared to go it alone.

In order to protect myself against these insidious and debilitating attacks of sabotage, which reinforce the onslaught of the virus, I'm sometimes tempted to start reasoning along the jingoistic lines of a Rea-

gan or a Rambo. I feel like one of those narrow-
minded diehards, and my America must believe in
itself to be strong, or else the enemy will take advantage of my moral weakness, distress, and the confusion I feel as a liberal intellectual caught in a
barbaric situation. The adventurism and superfi-
ciality of this kind of thinking would be dangerous
if I were to lose my sense of reality and overestimate
my own strength. The problem is that I'm not in
Hollywood, and the virus is not a cardboard mon-
ster. I mustn't panic and go to pieces, but instead
believe profoundly in my own values, which are
traditional to me even though they don't correspond
to those of the majority.

All these inner misgivings we feel about our ability
to survive constitute an entire syndrome, which I
call our Trojan horse, and we allowed this Trojan
horse within our gates long before the virus arrived
on the scene. It caused our first defeats, and merits
a special counterstrategy. Now, more than ever, we
are our own worst enemy, because we know our
own weaknesses so very, very well.

Like Birnam Wood in *Macbeth*, the epidemic
rushes onward to fulfill the prophecy of God's
wrath. Always ready to plead guilty, homosexuals
have decided that the virus, like those soldiers bearing tree branches, is the grotesque realization of
everything they had long dreaded would overtake
them. Cooler heads would never have managed to

persuade Macbeth that this forest on the march was only an army in camouflage; just try to convince people with AIDS that their virus is a virus like all the rest, even if it displays the unusual characteristics of a retrovirus (the medical terminology is somewhat ironic here). They all *know*, in their heart of hearts, that there is a more profound reality behind all these reasonable explanations: a punishment from heaven that will not be denied. They might just as well lay down their arms, faced with an enemy against which all weapons—and all defenses—are useless. If I could only demystify and exorcise the specter of AIDS, the way a soldier must learn to see only other men behind the fearsome mystery of the enemy!

Just as there are dirty wars, there are dirty diseases like AIDS that arouse no sympathy from the public, which prefers to shudder over them at a safe distance, without learning too many of the sordid details. The general opinion is that the epidemic is an obscure threat but, luckily, a remote one. In *Coming Home*, the soldier returning from Vietnam gets a chilly reception; he's suspected of having thrown away America's chance at victory by incapacitating himself through drug abuse and especially by living it up in Saigon. An AIDS patient is just as cruelly rebuffed if he confides in his family or colleagues. He quickly finds he has become a pariah, not necessarily because of an irrational fear of contagion, but through the instinctive revulsion felt for people stricken with misfortune. If even our leaders and doctors show that they have no faith in our courage or our moral and physical strength, how can we feel confident of victory? In the United States, most doctors are content with doing very little: it's enough for them to prolong this strange war by pretending to fight with the few traditional weapons at hand, but in so doing they risk courting an even more devastating defeat. I see so many comrades whose doctors have no real faith in their patients' survival and themselves may live in dread of the disease if they belong to a high-risk group.

Even more than our immunity, it's our confidence that the virus has destroyed. We no longer believe in ourselves, or in all those who have betrayed and deceived us. Like so many King Lears stripped of our illusions, we must wander blindly and alone, exposed to the bitter winds of doubt and suspicion.

HOPE RECAPTURED

FOR ME, AIDS was first of all the experience of solitude. Oliver's death and endless agony—which lasted only three months—quite naturally loosed all the ties that still bound me to the world of healthy people. Most of them would never have been able to understand what we went through, Oliver, his mother, and I, all three of us shut up in our space capsule, companions in misfortune on this nightmarish journey. Whenever I came home to a household completely disrupted by an invasion of medical technology, I wasn't sure whether I was landing on Mars or whether we were actually the only survivors of an atomic winter, abandoned by all our friends and colleagues—however compassionate—who had deserted our planet.

After Julia had gone, cradling in her lap an urn containing her son's ashes, I found myself alone on the front line.

This isolation must be my point of departure: I knew from that moment that I would die alone, and that I would endure my illness alone. If Oliver and I had struggled in vain to break down the barrier this disease had raised between us, who would be able to help me? We had become strangers to one another because I did not yet belong to his world of serious illness; I'd accompanied him as far as I could go, to the very threshold of death, but he had had to make his way through his last weeks of martyrdom alone.

To mourn for Oliver would have meant mourning for myself as well. By dying, he allowed me to live, releasing me from the burden of his survival, which had clearly brought me close to collapse that winter. At the time I couldn't imagine how I might bring him back safe and sound from the front line, airlifting him out of the jungle of AIDS. So Oliver decided at the appropriate moment to stop clinging to life. I don't know to what extent he was thinking of me when he made up his mind, with his mother's tacit consent, to unplug the machines around our bed that kept him alive through constant rehydration. I want to believe that he saw I still had a chance to escape from our camp on my own but that I'd never make it if, like Aeneas, I had to carry a frail old man's body on my back. I'll never freely admit that I hoped his end would come quickly, not only to release him from his agony but also to allow me to concentrate on my own survival. I'm tormented by guilt at having watched my own "partner"—to use my visiting nurse's discreet term—die in my place, tormented by the idea that he sacrificed himself not only for his mother but also for me, even though I try to convince myself that it really was the best thing for all concerned, as they say. My ally had become a liability. Like Amédée's relentlessly swelling corpse in Ionesco's play, his already ungainly body finally took up so much space in the loft that we had no room left to breathe. When the muffled wheezing of his respiration died away, when the heaving of his wasted rib cage ceased at last, my sobbing betrayed my cowardly relief.

Strangely enough, the very fact that we were both stricken with AIDS had come between us, because his illness progressed so much more rapidly than mine. I felt guilty for suffering less than he did, for still being able to take a space shuttle every day to go to my office and run the errands that provided us with food and medicine. I know that the contagious nature of AIDS has led to more and more couples having the disease and increased the number of households with AIDS, but in our case the illness cruelly divided us in life the better to strike us down, like the Curiatii.

My solitude was reinforced by my feeling that everything I read or observed in the media seemed so false, so pathetically at odds with my reality that I wondered if my sensory organs had somehow become different from everyone else's.

I was reliving "The Metamorphosis." I realized that my wing cases were frightening other people and that I would slowly cease to be a human being in their eyes, the Gregor Emmanuel Samsa they had always known. One day, they would ask the maid to come and sweep up my body and dump it in the garbage can. In short, I had passed Kafka's point of no return.

As the sole protagonist in my drama, with no one to talk to anymore, for the first time in my life I began keeping a diary, from which these pages have been drawn. From then on there were two of us—again, like Anne Frank. So, eager for even more company, I repopulated my universe with the only being whom I truly missed. I conjured up a complete puppet theater, a whole barracksful of toy soldiers, a voodoo exercise that did lead, in the end, to my emergence from the burrow where I'd gone to ground. I wasn't going to wait there any longer for AIDS to come and smoke me out. I found myself in the open air, clutching a submachine gun. It wasn't a hallucination: there really was an army all around me, an army whose existence I'd never even suspected. What follows is not a metaphor; it is an allegory, at most.

Since my doctors were of vital importance to me at that time, they were the first to be fitted out in the uniform of my army. I feel the same filial attachment to these men (Sonnabend and Kotler) that a simple soldier feels toward the leader of his regiment. I enjoy discussing their personality traits with other patients, just as Proust's Saint-Loup delighted in telling anecdotes about his commanding officer, the Prince de Borodino. The thing is that they're good leaders: Sonnabend knows how to show his humanity, how to reward the brave AIDS patient with a few words of encouragement and a conspiratorial wink: "You've gained four pounds this week!" He might almost have you believing that your progress is due to your own willpower and not to the effects of his medical treatment. The quality the troops value the most in their leaders is unpretentiousness: without demagogy, a superior officer makes each infantryman feel that no battle can ever be won without him. On the other hand, too many doctors favor a Prussian discipline, which obtains the same results from different patients, I must admit. Still, their attitude does lack that element of praise for the patient's personal accomplishment that is so important in maintaining his morale. Perhaps it's a question of temperament. In any case, I have the support I need to keep my spirits up and make me believe that I can win. Kotler, my gastrointestinal specialist, delivered a stirring speech to me yesterday on the increasing likelihood of therapeutic advances through transfusions (which would bring new blood to the front, healthy young recruits, like those fifteen-year-old soldiers in the Iranian Army). He told me I had to clench my teeth (and my buttocks, I suppose), square my shoulders, and look the enemy right in the eye. A real pep talk, like a general addressing the troops before Austerlitz. He talks about me on the phone to another patient under siege, telling him that my battalion is holding its own with the same medicine he has, thus encouraging my unknown comrade to take heart from my example.

My confidence in my superiors must be constantly reinforced by their sangfroid, because if I start questioning their decisions, I risk going into a tailspin. As it happens, like all those with AIDS in New York, I have at my disposal many sources of information on the latest tactics and therapies. In the lull between attacks, patients try to figure out the official line on their treatment from the apparent anarchy of commands and countermands issuing from headquarters, which possesses data we couldn't possibly interpret—at least in the first few months—even if we were privy to their information. Confidence in our chiefs is therefore essential, because if the doctor seems to be dodging the issue or losing interest in a particular symptom, or even worse, paying more attention to another case, another battalion, the AIDS patient loses ground and faith in his chances of holding on. Those who are most critical of their doctors—sometimes with good cause—are like soldiers embittered by their unwilling involvement in what they see as a senseless war, soldiers who complain constantly about the discomfort, privations, and risks of combat, never missing an opportunity to vent their hatred and impotent rage. This bitterness leads certain AIDS patients to alienate the very people who try to help them, so great is their resentment against the whole human race, especially those who weren't called up by AIDS and seem to enjoy insolent good health.

Unfortunately, I find myself coming up against Cassandras even among hospital personnel, who quite obviously think we're going to be not just decimated but completely wiped out, all of us, sooner or later. Even Dan, my visiting nurse, sincerely believes in the inevitability of defeat like everyone else. I know that I must follow his orders and let him decide on the dosage of my medicines and the schedule of my blood samples. Military hierarchy turns civilian social structures upside down, and strangers have suddenly become our superiors. Dan, a former fireman, risks his life by handling my blood specimens. He once told me that he soon learned to recognize which new recruits would die quickly and which ones had an instinct for survival.

Recently, with a mixture of pride and embarrassment, he brought me an article about the daily acts of charity he was performing as a nurse specialist assigned to outpatients like myself with AIDS. A quotation from him, printed as a caption beneath his photograph, sums up the message of the article: "They're all going to die." Dan feels that his role is to make our last few weeks less lonely and difficult. The first time I met him at the hospital, I knew that was how he saw things. He was already beginning each sentence with "sooner or later" and telling me that I would doubtless be stricken in succession by blindness, baldness, sterility, and finally death, which would be waiting for me at the end of my combatant's obstacle course, this deadly game of snakes and ladders. When Dan informed me that he had been made a special eucharistic minister in the Catholic Church, he pointed out that he would consequently be able to arrange for me to receive extreme unction. Our eternal salvation preoccupies him more than the number of our white blood cells. He doesn't really believe in my crazy dreams of getting well again: he thinks I'm just tilting at windmills.

So this virile and tutelary figure, who comes to my home twice a week to replenish my medical supplies and make sure that I'm following my instructions, is someone to whom I must prove my courage. When he inserts the intravenous catheter needle, I must grit my teeth (imagining, and why not, that I'm biting on a bullet) and pretend he's working on someone else's body. Certain soldiers back from the front line will admit that they often experienced a feeling of exaltation when they were in action, a sort of second state that they feel enables them to escape dangers against which reason alone would be helpless. They "knew" exactly when to crouch down or stand up, when to dodge bullets or adjust their aim. That's the state to which AIDS patients should aspire: to throw themselves so deeply into the struggle in which they are embroiled that pain and fear melt away, allowing better instincts to prevail over panic and despair. Fight, not flight.

THE TEMPTATION
OF DESERTION

THE IMPULSE TO DESERT recurs inevitably each time the illness tightens the screws a bit more. My intestinal war broke out again this week, and it's a constant worry to me. Judging from my previous experience with these bouts of diarrhea, I'm afraid I'm in for a bad time of it. The color, odor, and consistency of the feces are as distinctive as the different types of aircraft launched in a bombing raid by the enemy. Instead of an oven producing compact and solid fecal matter, like bricks baked in the sunshine of health, my guts have become a cesspool, a walking slop bucket full of nauseating gases and liquids, a tepid culture medium aswarm with the myriad amoebas and viruses of my personal chaos. The functioning—or, rather, the inertia—of my bowels is completely beyond my control. When I climb out of bed some mornings, I can almost hear myself sloshing, while "good days" find me holding firm, like a block of marble, with order temporarily restored. Discharges are always unconsciously feminizing, which doesn't help the martial image I try to have of myself.

Like successive waves of enemy soldiers advancing

to capture one of my positions, then falling back only to strike again with renewed fury, my diarrheas progress inexorably, undermining my morale and eating into my reserves. Panic ensues, spreading like wildfire when the enemy presses his advantage, when a lull in the battle suddenly erupts into fighting, and I must scramble to forestall a humiliating collapse on the sphincter front. Surprise attacks can strike all through the night, suddenly interrupting my rest with stomach-cramp flares. Still half asleep, I dash for the bathroom the way a soldier stupefied with fatigue runs for cover while reloading his gun, cursing the enemy for attacking like that at such an ungodly hour. The psychological effect of these raids can be devastating if the enemy launches three or four of them on the same night, especially if I have an "accident" before I can get to the blessed throne. The warrior's humiliation at being caught with his pants down is bad for morale; that's what happened to me today at dawn. I can't sleep naked anymore, the way I used to in peacetime. Now I wear my armor—underpants—at all times. Oliver was so harassed by the enemy that he even had to wear adult-size diapers.

The temptation to desert, to break out of the vicious circle of this dirty war, sometimes grabs me by the throat after a night like that. To slip out of Stalingrad, glimpse the countryside, be free of the German vise grip for only a moment; to escape in a balloon from besieged Paris, perhaps, like Gambetta in my elementary-school book; to experience that state of weightlessness without AIDS—a prisoner's dream, the fantasy of a soldier who knows full well that if he tried to desert, to abandon his treatment, he'd be shot by a firing squad on the spot: a dishonorable death and the sudden ruination of months of effort. And yet, how I understand him, the deserter overwhelmed by a pitiful lassitude. *Eli, Eli, lama sabachtani!* Oliver's prolonged and futile suffering was as heartrending as that of a young soldier gut-shot and abandoned by his comrades out on the battlefield. He would writhe in agony, livid, gripping his belly, his torment dragging on like that of Americans mortally wounded in the jungles of Vietnam, who would finally close their eyes, alone with death, convinced that the world had forgotten them, that they were dying for nothing. That's what the Jewish slave laborers in the camps thought too: the Gentile world had long since lost interest in their fate. Rounded up and transported, they had become invisible. Though I'm not one of those people who think that AIDS was created on purpose by someone somewhere, the fact remains that this epidemic was tolerated during at least the first two years by an entire society that believed itself safe from attack.

Is there any one of us who hasn't lived the nightmare of abandonment, those moments when we convince ourselves that the generals, medics, war correspondents, our companions in the struggle, our buddies will all forget us, have forgotten us, and are showing only the barest polite interest in our fight? Your wife will remarry; she's already cheating on you. That's when you long with all your heart, not for the wound that will invalid you out of the army, because you'll never get discharged, but for the bullet that will finish you off. How many have turned their weapons on themselves? Only their commanding officers could say, but they don't wish to demoralize the troops. There comes a moment when there's just no light at all at the end of the tunnel. If only I could throw away my weapon and go to meet the enemy, playing loud music to drown out the constant noise from the infusion pump at my bedside, which rattles when there's air trapped in the line. I don't know if I should talk about the siren call of defeatism, because the cynicism of a wounded AIDS veteran might upset the green recruits. Hadn't I better keep quiet instead of admitting that I sometimes think I'll never see the dawn of victory? What if I tossed all the medicines in my refrigerator out the window onto the heads of passersby, blew up my ammunition dump and supply depot, hopped into my jeep and drove it over a cliff shouting, "What the hell!" The ophthalmologist tells me that the cytomegalovirus is now present in my left eye, which had been healthy until now. Unable to vent my rage against any human being, I go home completely exasperated and start furiously kicking the doors and furniture; then, stymied by a recalcitrant can opener, I find myself screaming, a terrifying outburst, the desperate howl of a beast at bay. And so I shriek on, all by myself, witnessed only by the undaunted TV screen and the oh-so-worried face of Colonel North. Is he the kind of soldier who unconsciously inspires me, I who am just as ready to venture into illegality and improvise my own personal war? I hope not.

It's perhaps because of this sense of helplessness that certain AIDS victims have felt compelled to arrange every detail of their funerals beforehand, choosing the clothes they want to be buried in (something by Girbaud, Yamamoto, or Ralph Lauren?), full-dress uniform, as it were. The only shred of free will left to these demoralized men is their choice of wood for the casket and the size of the death announcement. Soldiers often confide their last wishes to their closest buddies, and give them things for safekeeping: letters to their mothers, cherished photographs with which they want to be buried. For a soldier, making these kinds of arrangements is less morbid and defeatist than it is for someone with AIDS; but doesn't the wholesale slaughter all around us justify such precautions?

Of course, most of us get a grip on ourselves in time. Even though cowardice may fascinate me for a moment and seek to push me into the abyss every few weeks, I naturally recover my equanimity. Actually, these morbid thoughts are perhaps as necessary as the daydreams of victory, of getting well again, those dreams evoked in such loving detail. You run through the list of everything you'll be able to do again—not necessarily in the sexual department, which is currently off-limits (life before the war, that inaccessible realm)—until a sudden cramp, like a grenade in the belly, wrenches you back to reality. The salutary opium of hypnotic reverie, when fingers relax on the trigger.

A ROMANTIC NIGHTMARE

ONLY THE MOST PERVERSE individuals, like me, can find AIDS romantic. Back when I still had ARC, or AIDS-related complex (the equivalent of adolescence when compared to my present mature AIDS manhood), I naïvely imagined the heroic glory of the patients at La Salpêtrière in Paris, those apparently healthy men who would tell me about the pneumonia they'd had six months before or show me the lesions on their legs.

I remember the mysterious aura I bestowed upon pioneer patients. Three years ago, at a brunch with friends who had AIDS, I couldn't help feeling elated at the sight of all those martyrs eating quiche and drinking tea, as though they didn't understand that they were enjoying only a temporary stay of execution—which was how I saw things at the time. To me, the daily life of an AIDS patient was as incomprehensible as that of the nobles imprisoned in La Conciergerie during the Terror, who had to go on washing, shaving, tending to their natural functions in a strange and frightening place. I didn't know what to talk about with these men: should I ask them to recount their war experiences or start chatting about the latest film? A man on leave doesn't need to say anything: he already commands respect from anyone with a bit of imagination. He'll be returning to the front after a brief respite that must seem quite unreal to him. His apparent calm is in fact heroic. A soldier can never stand at ease and must display the signs of his heroism with the regularity of a nervous tic. Since being sent to the front myself, I've come to understand the banality of the everyday courage demanded by the situation, that simple lack of any other possible response, aside from madness or suicide.

Every army has its daredevils, and I used to dream unconsciously of wounds and bruises. I longed to enlist, almost as though I wanted to beat the draft by joining up. I was also worried about how I would react at meeting the enemy for the first time, when I encountered my first opportunistic illness. Obviously, my body's response was a source of some concern to me, but my mental attitude preoccupied me even more. Would I be a coward? Would I accept without flinching the wounds and amputations that so often accompany the evolution of the disease? In a sense, it would be better if my corpse could resemble that of Rimbaud's Sleeper in the Valley, so untouched by death that only by bending low over him could one see the blood welling up from "two red holes on his right side." Unfortunately, AIDS doesn't offer that option to narcissistic homosexuals, eating away at them instead with its little rat teeth, covering their bodies and faces with its ivy, gripping them in such a stranglehold that the more the victims struggle in their terror, the tighter they are held, until they lie at last under an oxygen tent that prolongs their sufferings in the trap. There are few Sleepers in the Valley in the armies of AIDS. At the very least, when I finally close my eyes it won't be with a bullet in the back, because it's pathetic to turn away from one's own death. The fact of being unable to look death in the face increases the feeling of panic that routs armies and kills the slightest impulse to fight back. I used to think that dying in one's sleep was a blessing, but now I would rather be in the highest state of awareness and intelligence when I experience that supreme flash of lightning.

I admit that I sometimes enjoy the admiration my martial attitude arouses in those close to me, and I'll take a certain pleasure in humming and whistling in public or grinning widely to make my audience think: "How brave he is . . ." It tickles me all the more to do this when I don't like the person I'm trying to impress, or when that person appears to doubt the possibility of victory. I'd rather seem unconscious of my danger than defeated by it. I'm well aware of the affectations that spring from my fear. I try to hide my moments of weakness and the effort it costs me to appear to lead a normal life, but when my public occasionally seems a trifle lacking in intuition, I'll discreetly bring my suffering to their

attention with a casual remark intended to reveal
the abyss of pain heroically concealed by my un-
ruffled demeanor. Thus hoping to arouse and maintain their interest, to inspire both pity and
admiration, I score on all counts. That's probably
what I'd do if I really went to war. I wouldn't complain, but I'd let fall—oh, quite involuntarily!—
some fleeting hint of both the horrors of the battlefield and the blushing modesty of my courage.

I consciously use blackmail to get what I want,
thereby following the dictates of the only morality
I respect: that of my own survival. If I write to
editors or literary agents, I never fail to slip in some
reference to the constraints my illness places on me,
some allusion to the inestimable value each passing
day has for me from now on. Do not an author and
a dying man both suffer the same torments? For
those close to me, my requests are often like dis-
guised commands. Some of us are tempted to ex-
aggerate the gravity of our situation to satisfy our
whims. Like a spoiled child, I let it be understood
that soon I'll have departed this life—and then they'll
be sorry!—which makes all the healthy "grown-ups"
feel guilty about standing safely on solid ground
watching me sink into quicksand. And they give in.
My favorite expression as a child, or so I've been
told, was "I've got my rights!" AIDS has given me
every right, like those crippled veterans who use
parking spaces "Reserved for the Disabled." I can

sense that my audience loses interest whenever my health seems to stabilize for a few weeks. That's when I suspect my unconscious of setting me up for a few bouts of diarrhea or some psychosomatic symptoms that will revive flagging sympathy and produce a flourish of handkerchiefs. This war of nerves is even more distressing for those who love me. Perhaps the situation shouldn't drag on forever: even the compassionate sister of the insect in "The Metamorphosis" finally tires of humoring him. When Richard, who later found me a publisher in the United States, told me that he sincerely hoped that my book would be translated and published "in your lifetime," I discovered that this image of a race against time was a reality for most people who come in contact with me. When I'm with Steve, another AIDS patient, we like to pick up on each other's careless remarks hinting at the inevitable deterioration of our health.

Other people's pity irritates me, but at the same time I need to have it, I'm hooked on it, and it helps justify my occasional episodes of self-pity. Why was I chosen, called up by AIDS, instead of my friends, my enemies, the masses of indifferent people who actually fit the same profile as I do, with lifestyles and even sexual habits that qualify them for the draft? Other people's enlistment seems more natural and logical to me than my own. I might almost say that they actively signed up, while I got press-ganged, perhaps through some computer error. In the beginning, when I had only passing malaises, intermittent fevers, swollen and aching lymph nodes, I still hoped that the bad test results were some mechanical or human mistake, that the whole thing was a ghastly misunderstanding. Life, alas, confirmed my call-up notice, and the first symptoms fitted me out with my helmet, combat boots, and knapsack for basic AIDS training. From now on I must rely above all on self-discipline to achieve the impossible, without daring to mention my ambition to get well again (that five-star general's cap), a naïve hope that would arouse only condescending or indulgent smiles from my friends. I feel torn between a feeling of spontaneous solidarity with my companions in misfortune and a barely concealed desire to get out of the front lines, obtain a deferment for good conduct, or be transferred to a less dangerous post.

I've recently discovered in myself a hitherto unsuspected interest in war films, which have given me useful lessons in keeping my sense of perspective: though I may sometimes venture out into the unknown, I've never had to advance against an intelligent and crafty enemy, as real soldiers do. I don't have to keep calmly lobbing grenades while my comrades get their insides or their brains blown to bits before my very eyes. During the Klaus Barbie trial in Lyons, the testimony of the tortured Jews and

Resistance fighters showed me that there was one dimension still lacking—fortunately—in my martial metaphor: pain, the kind of torment that brings you to your knees, robs you of your dignity, drags you down to the level of an animal. I know that I would have spilled my guts, told them absolutely everything at the mere sight of the torture chamber. My illness seems to have kept this weapon in reserve and only rarely forces me to admit that I'm completely at its mercy. Others aren't as lucky as I am: they feel the iron grip of the disease crushing their lungs, twisting their entrails. No tranquilizer can dispel their splitting headaches; no lotion can soothe the ferocious itching of the lesions festering on their bodies. In their situation, with an illiterate brute twisting my arm like that, I'd never have been able to write a single line.

Our enemy is using live ammunition, there's no doubt about that, but the panic I sometimes feel when I wake up from a bad dream, for example, isn't as terrifying as the fear that enveloped soldiers fighting in Vietnam. Those of us with AIDS kill no other human beings except our former selves. We'll never shed anyone else's blood. My recurring nightmares, at least the ones I can remember, all have to do with my doctors and medicines. I once dreamed that one of my intravenous drug pouches was filled with a dark, reddish-brown liquid instead of the usual transparent fluid, but my nurse kept reassuring me that it was all right for me to put this substance in my veins. When I finally gave in, I awoke bathed in sweat. And I've been waking up like that every morning for the past few months, whatever the reason. Soldiers must also have disturbing dreams, in which they're threatened and deceived by their own officers or the enemy. Paradoxically, when I open my eyes and look around at all the hospital equipment by my bed, I still think: "Well, it was just a nightmare. I've only got AIDS and I'm not trapped in all that horror I was dreaming about." Isn't a soldier similarly relieved to find, when he awakens, that it's only war out there, and not his own, even more terrible, hallucinatory universe? How can I find rest at night when I'm under such pressure, day after day, month after month? Soldiers go on having war dreams for years after the fighting is over; my unconscious will always be marked by AIDS, if I ever get over it. I'll never be able to see a hypodermic without thinking of "it," or hear the word "diapers" without remembering Oliver's skeletal body in those adult swaddling clothes, like a bulky, rustling pair of rompers. For me, the neighborhood around St. Luke's Hospital is like one of those innocent fields of vegetables near Verdun that evoke memories of terrible bloodshed only in the soldiers who once fought there for months. Thousands of dead and wounded have passed that way, leaving an indelible mark visible only to me and my fellow AIDS patients.

I'm also visited almost every evening by my lost companion, killed in action before his time. I struggle so furiously during the night against these imaginary enemies, about whom I don't dare think in my waking hours, that by morning my pillows and blankets are scattered all over the floor, leaving me shivering without so much as a sheet to protect me from my nocturnal visitors. My bed winds up so rumpled that it suggests prolonged erotic acrobatics when in fact I've simply been defending myself, like Monsieur Seguin's poor goat. I was traumatized as a child by Alphonse Daudet's story, and profoundly disturbed by its sad conclusion. When I first read the tale I was still accustomed to Hollywoodian happy endings, so I expected the goat to survive the wolf's attack after having fought him off all night long. It was only logical to assume that she would be saved and rewarded by the arrival of Monsieur Seguin in the morning. And yet the unhappy animal seems to have fought in vain, since she finally surrenders, panting with exhaustion, at sunrise. I was so angry with the author for having refused the easy way out and for having tried to teach me to fight for the principle of the thing, to preserve my dignity, whatever the outcome might be. The AIDS wolf and General Franco may win in the end, but what counts is fighting honorably at Madrid or withstanding the siege at St. Luke's. That's when one turns to one's childhood heroes, like the frontier woodsman Davy Crockett, the man who knew no fear. He could beat the Indians at their own game and waged his personal war in a strange new world. Like a trapper, I must learn to recognize the tracks of each opportunistic illness and adapt myself to the material conditions of the moment, however difficult they may be—a stay in the hospital, a sleepless night, the insertion of a new catheter—whistling all the while in the chilly solitude of that dark forest where I wander without hope of ever finding a sympathetic Virgil.

SANS GOD, SANS MEN

THOSE WHO BELIEVE in heaven and those who don't all share the same faith in the fight against AIDS. I can't help envying patients who believe in the efficacy of prayer and their right to call upon divine justice for help in overcoming this trial. Julia prays for me every day, and Frank's mother does too, the way a soldier's mother will place a photograph of her hero near a statue of the Virgin and kneel before it. I've even renounced my former Voltairean hostility to such things, so that when Scott told me he was praying for me, at a time when everything seemed to be going badly and my front line appeared in danger of collapsing, I gratefully accepted his spiritual reinforcement instead of sneering at him like a radical atheist. Many priests and nuns accompany soldiers as close as possible to the enemy lines, and army chaplains are sometimes killed in action along with the rest of the men. Some priests have already died of AIDS, while others, although wounded, manage to continue their ministry, unless they're forced out of their congregations as traitors.

The hostility of religious leaders toward those who have AIDS poses an additional threat to patients who are believers: the preachers of the Moral Majority condemn them outright before millions of television viewers and call more or less openly for their destruction. A bit like Pope Pius XII blessing Mussolini's planes as they prepared to take off on bombing raids over the strongholds of republican loyalists in Spain—many of whom were fervent Catholics. AIDS patients don't receive the moral support they're entitled to expect from their churches and particularly from the higher religious authorities, who maintain an attitude of prudent neutrality since they don't consider many AIDS victims to be good Christians deserving of God's mercy in their moment of trial. This reproving and vindictive God who is supposed to have visited his biblical wrath upon our Sodom is also something of a Trojan horse, since he's the foe of the besieged, as Athena was at Troy: once admitted into the religious convictions of those ill with AIDS, this wrathful God weakens their resistance by making them doubt the justice of their cause. In every conflict (unless one of the warring nations is Communist and atheistic), each antagonist has claimed God for its side, the French as well as the Germans, the members of Dignity as well as the bishops of Manhattan and Brooklyn, who want to prevent any homosexual group—whether or not its members have AIDS—from meeting in their churches. Chaplains in the French and German armies told their countrymen that their cause was righteous and beloved of God. I hope that history will deal harshly with all pastors who betrayed those in their spiritual care. The Vatican has always managed to make it through a war with seemingly clean hands, even though its image was somewhat tarnished by the papal silence during the period of Nazi terror. There were anti-Semites in the Church in those days just as there are homophobic priests now, priests who turn away from AIDS sufferers appealing to them at the eleventh hour, deny them sanctuary, and leave them to be massacred by the enemy at their very doorstep. Will the Church go so far as to erect a monument, another Sacré-Coeur to celebrate our destruction? In their eyes we are rebellious Communards and the basest of libertines. The Pope, for one, seems to feel that the moral and edifying principles of the Bible take precedence over the humanitarian forgiveness of the Gospel.

A friend who is interested in mysticism has advised me to follow his example and seek serenity in India, in the ashram of his guru, not in order to regain my health, but to prepare myself for death, or so I suppose. He simply cannot understand why I insist on remaining in New York. It's just that I don't see myself as a pure soul already detached from this world of ours. I'm deeply attached to reality, and my spiritual salvation could not possibly exclude my support group, those who take care of and care about me. And think how many diseases I would be exposing myself to in India, diseases that would merely hasten my death. The only comfort I might find there would be the realization that my life as an AIDS patient in New York would seem enviable to the beggars lined up at the temple gates, silently displaying their pustules and withered limbs. No: my salvation must come from within.

It was Michel Tournier's conceit that Gilles de Rais turned to a life of crime and debauchery after witnessing Joan of Arc being burned at the stake in Rouen. As for me, I hope to emerge victorious by transforming myself into the Maid of Orléans and burning my former incarnation as Gilles de Rais. At the time, they said that France had been lost by a whore, Isabeau de Bavière, and would be saved by a virgin. So I'm counting on driving the enemy out of my kingdom with the help of the archangels—the same ones invoked by Proust's Baron de Charlus in the twilight of his life—who will surely take an interest in my new incarnation. Was I unknowingly thinking along those lines when I decided to give up any further sexual contacts? I suspect the primitive and superstitious medieval peasant in me of having tacitly concluded such a pact. If a simple country girl was able to address the king of France, take command of an army, and liberate Orléans, then I should be able to obtain at least a remission using the same approach. Thanks to my rediscovered virginity.

What many young homosexuals of the prewar period found particularly exciting in their sexual activity was its anonymity: the fact that one didn't know one's partner made him all the more desirable, and the impersonality of the places where one met was precisely what made these surroundings seem supercharged with sexuality. I felt that in their search for pleasure these young men were unconsciously looking for "foreigners" whom they could "shoot," finding such pursuits easier and more exhilarating than a love relationship with a familiar partner. These days the situation is reversed, and those who still lead an active sexual life are looking instead for comrades, partners in whom they can have confidence and whose medical history is well known to them. Since any friend or lover may now prove to be an "enemy," it's less exciting to go out looking for strangers. The danger implicit in all sexual acts for thousands of years has just been made concrete by this virus, a far more serious threat than the pathetic venereal diseases of yesteryear, those battles waged with blowguns and catapults. Anonymity and promiscuity are also two themes in war literature: men who are complete strangers to one another must live and die side by side, in an intimacy that is often initially quite embarrassing, almost obscene. Our present combat is a new Dance of Death that continues relentlessly no matter how many of us fall by the wayside. Some militant AIDS patients hope to make use of the collective energy we used to expend in our quasi-tribal sexuality to launch a modern Crusade. All the veterans of our persuasion would join this new order of chivalry uniting those homosexuals who are still healthy and those who have already been knighted by AIDS. Ideally, our vanguard should encourage all Americans to band together against this absolute evil.

After I was diagnosed as having AIDS during a bout of pneumonia, it took me more than a year to give up being sexually active, to renounce the pleasures of the flesh, inch by inch, and learn to practice a monkish abstinence. I've become as chaste as a Crusader, or a knight on the eve of combat, those warriors who sublimated sexual energy in love of country and ardor on the battlefield. My decision is obviously due to circumstances beyond my control. Who would agree to be my partner, knowing of my condition? How could I dare let anyone see this body of which I was once proud and which now, through lack of exercise, has become a potbellied puppet with scrawny limbs whose flesh has melted away in the searing furnace of AIDS? The average foot soldier in our army hardly corresponds to the courtly ideal and isn't likely to satisfy anyone except thrill seekers excited by the rank odor of big game.

As it happens, I'd smell more like the chlorine I use to disinfect everything or the alcohol with which I clean my catheter before each shot.

Soldiers at the front have their traditional pen pals, their mothers and fiancées, venerated icons of purity—at least according to the official version of these things—even though they may occasionally go off to a brothel to party with whores, whom they despise. Last summer, for example, the few safe-sex encounters I experienced were hardly distinguishable—even though they weren't venal transactions—from the impersonal relations between prostitutes and their clients. I was looking only for superficial contact, skin contact, and the setting I chose was as anonymous as possible. This sex on the run, snatched during a lull in the action, is the only option available to people with AIDS who live alone and have no lovers. For homosexuals, the army was traditionally a well-stocked preserve of men left on their own who might possibly be tempted by forbidden fruit while temporarily cut off from women. In the war against AIDS, homosexuality in itself is dangerous because it's the loaded weapon pointing at our own bodies, the bayonet thrust into our emaciated and now undesirable loins. I don't worship at the altar of sex anymore, as the sting of death is much more fascinating.

A soldier in action forgets all about sex as long as he's kept busy just trying to stay alive, but occasionally, in the bleakest moments, he may turn to erotic fantasies to ward off fear or lull himself to sleep. I've so many other things to worry about now that my sexual frustration is a fairly minor problem, whereas I used to be quite highly sexed. The time for sexual extravagance is past, and now seems rather futile confronted with the majesty of death. The media and the public are naturally fascinated by the bond AIDS establishes between sex and death, that copulation between the two most effect-laden primitive forces, now forever linked in people's minds with homosexuals. One example of this association is the controversy over whether or not to close the bathhouses in San Francisco, but I don't see that it really poses a problem of freedom of choice. To me, these last bastions of our former sexuality represent places where energies needed for the war effort are— or would be—simply wasted. The sexual hard core still frequenting them feels a certain sense of failure, whatever they may say, over their inability to give up their prewar attitudes and promiscuity. In addition, society's enemy propaganda seizes on such things to launch outraged attacks on these individuals and the entire gay community through retroactive or collective guilt, considering such "dens of iniquity" to be seething cauldrons spreading all the germs and viruses released by the Pandora's box of nature and the sexual revolution. The baths aren't

like brothels frequented by soldiers, but rather resemble another Trojan horse, this one a miserable
nag like Don Quixote's Rocinante. In my halluci-
nations this animal collapses in a last spasm on its
equally emaciated partner and adversary.

My doctor is of the liberal school. In the interests
of bolstering the morale of AIDS patients, he feels
justified in permitting them to have safe physical
contacts, even encouraging them in this direction.
I refuse to go to those social gatherings, sponsored
by sympathizing organizations, for lonely AIDS patients looking for partners, even though I know
some people who have gone on dates this way. I'm
too obsessed with my private battle. Like a gunner
fascinated by his machine, I'd rather spend my evenings studying ballistics and the enemy's tactics instead of going to the officers' club to drink and talk
about women. Perhaps I'm deluding myself with
the idea that by making an offering of my body,
virtuous once more (at least in deed), I will manage
to satisfy the Beast and thus reach the opposite shore
unscathed. I won't remarry until after the Libera-
tion, when there'll be no more risk that my partner
might turn out to be one of the enemy. In the mean-
time, my armor must be kept shining and spotless,
unstained by the slightest trace of sperm or body
fluids. I must be as one dead to my passions in order
to triumph and reestablish concord between body

and soul: that is my motto. Preparation for a holy war is not simply a question of physical training; it's an introduction to the mystical life through asceticism. I should aspire to be wedded to health in a spiritual union, like that of St. Theresa of Avila with Christ, thus achieving sainthood. Actually, my only intercessor is my wavering faith in medicine, Aesculapius, that god who sometimes cuts a pretty miserable figure.

Like Achilles without Patroclus, naturally I envy—relatively speaking—those AIDS patients who are partners in a loving relationship. Like officers with special permission to live and travel with their wives, they can enjoy their lovers' moral support, and in the best of cases even their sexual availability, which makes the break with their pre-AIDS lives less traumatic. They have someone close to them urging them to cling to life and win the battle for both their sakes. They're like Spartan warriors, a regiment of lovers. The Trojans in their besieged city had the same advantage: at nightfall, binding up their husbands' wounds, the women of Troy would praise their courage and increase their determination to resist the enemy, which they did for twenty years—AIDS patients aren't asking for that much time—while the Greeks camped out in tents, without the comfort of their wives and families. Helen was waiting night after night to welcome Paris home with open arms, giving him fresh reasons to fight again the following day, and I like to think that the lovers of people with AIDS treat their companions with redoubled tenderness.

Encouraged by this emotional bond, by this constant reminder of the attractions of homosexual life, a patient thus cared for draws strength from his sexual patriotism.

The majority of AIDS victims, however, suffer the sexual misery of ostracism. Once the lights and the television are turned off at night, panic sets in, and the slow, monotonous, but reassuring ritual of masturbation reminds us of the time when we wandered without a care in the crimson paradise of sexuality. More than a kind of tranquilizer, masturbation is a way we young men have of escaping for a short time from the prisonlike world in which we're trapped by the horror we inspire in others. Any military campaign may harbor unscrupulous soldiers who rape defenseless women when they get the chance; people with AIDS who don't tell their partners that they're sick and don't take any precautions are doing the same thing. I feel the same contempt for them that West Pointers feel for the soldiers involved in the My Lai massacre. I suspect those renegades of wanting to make all civilians pay for their good luck and their indifference. They must feel so much hatred for themselves and everyone else!

In the case of homosexual AIDS patients, the sexual origin of the disease increases our distress and confusion. Not only do we find ourselves suddenly uprooted from everything dear to us, but from now on we must also fear and distrust one of our traditional refuges. Before the epidemic, we often turned to sex to relieve the depression we sometimes felt; there were those who maintained, ten years ago, that an evening in a bathhouse was worth weeks of therapy. Now even this comfort is denied us at the very moment when we've been hurled into the immense solitude of AIDS.

THE WAR ZONE
AND THE HOME FRONT

TORN FROM OUR FAMILIAR surroundings, we feel our exile even more poignantly in the hospitals, our "trenches," places as repulsive to us as those endless labyrinths of mud where our grandfathers floundered in the grip of World War I. These hospitals are like so many war zones from which civilians have been evacuated, where all movement is strictly controlled and limited, where only those with special passes are allowed to come anywhere near our illness. This image comes to mind because people with AIDS are isolated and kept in quarantine, unlike patients with cancer or other diseases. Only specialists and courageous friends and relatives who obtain the proper authorization are permitted to visit us. All these barriers set up between areas of health and areas of AIDS accentuate our solitude, because we can still see, through the barbed wire, how those in the unoccupied zone go on about their lives as usual.

When I arrived at St. Luke's Hospital, I understood immediately why some people love the army: they're relieved to know that all responsibility for their fate has been taken out of their hands. Hospitalized patients find themselves in the same situation as soldiers; they're required to wear uniforms, expected to obey all orders, and subjected to absurd rules (they would wake me at six in the morning, to weigh me and take my temperature, after which I was supposed to go back to sleep until nine). Life in barracks and hospitals is a constant rhythm of people going on duty, coming off duty, arriving on schedule with the meal carts loaded with trays, and so forth. The first thing they gave me at St. Luke's was a copy of the hospital rules announcing the militarization of my conduct. I was forbidden to leave the floor, smoke, drink, gamble, and so forth. All these instructions are not so much for the good of the patient or his country as for the benefit of the institution, be it hospital or army, and they are designed to erase our personalities, so is it any wonder that individual victories are so rare? It's true that many patients prefer to die according to the rules of medicine, to paraphrase Molière, instead of living by disobeying them. They remind me of those commanders who elect to lose a war fighting by the book instead of winning by taking a chance on innovative military strategy. As soon as I arrived, I made a point of furnishing my room with books and other familiar objects, and I refused to put on that ridiculous hospital gown they have in America, which I find humiliating because it opens down the back and thus can't be fastened without the help of a nurse. I wore my own clothes in my room, putting on my AIDS uniform only when I had to go for tests in another wing of the hospital, a trip I was always obliged to make in a wheelchair and wearing a perfectly useless surgical mask just to reassure the hospital attendant on transport detail.

Given the number and seriousness of the opportunistic diseases clustered around AIDS, a patient may stay a long time, sometimes indefinitely, in the same hospital room. After a few days in mine, I had completely lost my sense of time. The telephone enabled me to keep in contact with the home front, where people were concerned about how I was doing and eager to send me special treats to perk up the usual dull hospital fare. I noticed that discipline tended to be either strict or relaxed from one shift to another, depending on the personality of the doctor in charge. On a different floor of the hospital, I wouldn't have been allowed to improvise my own uniform, because the "warrant officer" there would have been much less flexible than mine. Like a soldier watching the passage of the seasons at Verdun, I literally saw the last snowflakes fall and the first tiny buds open from the same window during my stay in the hospital. In an adjoining room, a black AIDS patient, probably an ex-junkie—but how could I be sure from what little I could see through the half-open door?—was breathing noisily in an oxygen mask, with the precious cylinder installed at his bedside. The virus had thrown a poison-gas grenade into his foxhole. During the long nights I spent in the hospital, lulled by this intermittent humming, I'd find myself staying on the qui vive, lying in wait for the shadowy forms that might appear on the enemy lines, anxious not to be caught off guard. A sudden râle from my neighbor would alert me at my sentry post.

I was vaguely aware that I couldn't always count on the hospital personnel. Certain nurses were openly afraid or hostile, and they reminded me of Nazi allies forcibly conscripted for service in occupied Europe. They took pains to let me know that this war wasn't their affair. I'm proud of having learned at the hospital how to administer my own treatment against CMV: I can load the three "machine guns" that I insert every day into the outside opening of my peripheral catheter, and I can operate the pump—real state-of-the-art technology—that shoots the antiviral reinforcements of DHPG, or ganciclovir, into my veins. What does it matter if these impedimenta hamper my mobility, as though I were a Roman foot soldier lugging around tools and armor? I've lost my former freedom of movement, but I try to think of myself as a true guerrilla, still independent, still managing on my own. The day Veronica came to get me at the hospital, the sunshine seemed even more beautiful to me because I knew I had made it through two grueling weeks on the front line. I was going home, crossing snowy Central Park in a taxi alive with tropical music. Ice skaters were venturing out onto the frozen lake. I felt like laughing out loud from the simple joy of having survived, of returning to my semi-civilian life. The taxi driver had picked me up like any other passenger. No longer would I be confined to a room with a door covered with warning signs, or surrounded by nurses and aides wearing gloves and masks, noting their observations in my file plastered with red circles and stickers reading: PRECAUTIONS—AIDS. In short, I was discharged and going home on a frosty day, on leave for what I hoped would be a very long time.

It may seem paradoxical to view the hospital as both a refuge and a battlefield, or my going home as both a discharge from active service and a return to the front. In the jumbled universe I've concocted for myself to rationalize my situation, however, I have no trouble accepting these contradictions. Everything has become ambiguous since I myself have lost my own ambivalence. Now, New York and life in general seem all the more desirable to me because I thought they were gone forever, like a fiancée whose charms are multiplied by the thought that one might never see her again. My hospitalization was a sanctuary, a period of calm that enabled me to restore certain defenses breached by the latest viral attack, then prudently reconnoiter the situation and even consider retaking a bit of lost ground, by regaining some weight and getting rid of the depressing circles under my eyes.

Daily life is another trial, and the dilemma is the same: Am I healthy or sick? Should I live normally or lie low, hibernating the way I'm inclined to do? In fact, I'm paralyzed by anxiety at having my life in my own hands: whatever decision that is mine alone to take—be it skipping a meal, taking a long bike ride, going to bed late—may well, in my symbolic universe, start me down the frightful toboggan run of AIDS. That's when I have to clutch at the slightest straw of reality to keep from losing my head. In a sense, I play at living, at going to the office, seeing films, joining friends in a restaurant, the way I used to play grocer or doctor, not far from Nasser's tanks when I was a child in Cairo. I pretend there's nothing wrong: balancing my checkbook regularly, paying electricity bills, making an appointment with the plumber for next Friday, repainting the kitchen, or buying books I may never get to read—especially if the CMV starts acting up again in my eyes.

This parody of normalcy is all the more pitiful when we must share festive moments with others, particularly when they themselves aren't sick. The illness really brings a new luster to occasions traditionally celebrated with friends or family. Christmas, Thanksgiving, and birthdays are given poignant new meaning by our tragic circumstances. Perhaps it was also like this in the concentration camps, this return of symbolic dates bringing with them the inevitable memories of happier times, before the shadow of death loomed over us. This nostalgia isn't necessarily for a childhood long past, because the dearest memories, and thus the saddest, are sometimes the most recent. Just before the declaration of war, people were still making plans for life as usual while the radios gave constant news coverage on Nuremberg rallies and the parliamentary debates over the German chancellor's ultimatums. Bored listeners would simply flip the dial to a station playing light music. Today, when AIDS is mentioned on television, many of us turn our stereos up a little louder and continue talking about our costumes for the next "Black Party" at The Saint.

I can't forget the sight of Oliver at a Thanksgiving dinner organized by kind neighbors, sitting with his mother on their last outing together, two weeks before his death. He, stiff and silent, with all the dignity of his twenty-four years and six feet two inches, doubtless comparing the happy Thanksgivings of his past with this quasi-parody hosted by semi-strangers with good intentions, but forced upon him by dismal circumstances. There was his mother, worried and attentive, but eager to experience a hint of the warmth of family meals gone

by. What a humiliating travesty, what an empty celebration that party was; our invalid couldn't touch
a single bite of the feast, as his digestive system had
long since ceased to function. Unable to eat, sad at
heart, he simply smiled sweetly at the civilians pretending for his benefit that everything was just fine
and being so careful not to mention the war raging
all around them. An artificial truce. At the hospital
as well, the usual bland menu is a bit fancier on
Christmas Day, and the muffled echoes of other
people's parties reach the patient lying in his dark-
ened room, watching the standardized TV version
of those holidays he can no longer experience for
himself.

I prefer to consider these occasions of obligatory
merrymaking as ordinary days like all the others, but
I put too much effort into my indifference for it to
be truly honest. In times of crisis, we try to cope
with fear by pretending that life goes on as usual,
by cooking a traditional meal or buying new clothes
for Easter. These dates are like crutches for our emotional life, and they take us back to the days of our
lost health. Every symbol counts in an existence as
artificial as that of a serious invalid, and they still
anchor us to reality, to the way the rest of society
lives. And so we're reassured to find that we still
belong to humanity, something we may occasionally
doubt when every day we come up against the horror—even the hatred—we inspire in healthy people,

who probably think they belong to some superior race. The Aryans of immunity.

Just as Proust's narrator saw his familiar bedroom transformed by his magic lantern into a place of mystery by the images projected onto the doorknob and the folds of the window curtains, so this illness casts a disquieting light over the humblest details of my life and the universe I thought I knew so well. Everything is new and strange to us, and we must reaccustom ourselves to reality as though we were young Mowglis, wild children abandoned in the jungle. My virgin forest is in Manhattan. Here in America, most people with AIDS live in or near a city, and I associate AIDS with the sidewalks of New York and San Francisco. As a city dweller with AIDS, I feel doubly out of place when I venture into the woods of upstate New York, where nature is quite indifferent to my struggle. At least I'm not a frightening intruder there: neither the dog nor the birds nor the plants tremble when they see me coming. And yet this bucolic setting, in which I only pretend to live, is merely a painted backdrop without real depth, like the sets in a German Expressionist movie. Since even our own bodies risk becoming strange to us, we must learn to resist the temptation to see them as hated antagonists. An AIDS patient must never forget that his body is his sole ally and reason for fighting, ungrateful though it may seem. We must learn to tame Bagheera.

Sometimes a question flashes through my mind
like a flare bursting in the night sky, and I wonder:
"What the fuck am I doing here?" Why have I agreed
to live out this nightmare? For one moment, I have
the illusion that I need only *want* to be well again
and I will be cured, a magic ending to this artificial
war, a return to the reality enjoyed by all those civilians around me. Because the overwhelming prospect of the talents and potential of an entire
generation of young people going to waste is simply
unreal. King Ubu has taken over my life. His diktats
are as extraordinary as the mobile infusion pump
that dominates my living room. I have to hook myself up to this contraption every day, which must
look rather bizarre, as if a guerrilla fighter were to
camp out on the parquet of a cozy bourgeois apartment, still clutching his machine gun. Now I don't
find it at all unusual to be suddenly on familiar terms
with strangers who proceed to tell me their life stories in detail, including their former sexual habits,
as soon as we discover we have the same kind of
diarrhea from the same kind of parasite. With my
respiratory problems, climbing up the six floors to
my apartment is another novel experience: I'm not
even forty yet and I'm learning what it's like to be
old. I feel like a busy city suddenly plunged into
darkness, forced to submit to a curfew by the threat
of enemy bombers. During the blackouts of the
Great War, Paris in the moonlight reminded Proust

of Baghdad, but my feeling of unreality is unfortunately rooted in something less enchanting than *The Arabian Nights*. Death—the incongruity of its presence in our still young lives—is the height of absurdity: it makes a mockery of all my efforts to continue to live normally despite its constant threat.

Other people's deaths don't affect us as much as they once did. The first victims were terrifying, and we meditated for a long time on their fate, their physical decay, their stoicism. Then, as the body count rose inexorably, we reached a kind of saturation point, when death simply became a part of our lives. In Roland Dorgelès's war novel *Les Croix de bois*, the soldiers buttress the walls of their trenches with the rotting corpses of their fallen comrades. Seasoned invalids learn to wear the same psychological armor, and thus may watch their best friends die without allowing themselves to lose heart. Every day, patiently, the corrosive power of habit turns death into a commonplace, and we become accustomed to the stink of charnel houses. The clamorous tributes paid—among ourselves—to our fallen in the first heroic days of combat have given way to hasty ceremonies before the common grave that daily swallows up dozens of corpses, tossed in pell-mell, as at the vast World War I cemetery of Douaumont. My inurement to the death of young people—AIDS patients are so often young—extends to the deaths of other generations, and other patients, and accident victims . . . in short to the death of any human being.

My unconscious reasons like primitive man, who cannot believe in the inevitability of his own death, which is excluded from his universe. My "considered" understanding of the risk of mortality is derived more from the information forced upon me by the media than it is from personal contacts, since the loss of this or that friend or acquaintance can always be attributed to bad luck, the ignorance of his doctors, an unfortunate set of circumstances, or the refusal to believe oneself ill or in danger, a refusal that many young AIDS patients obstinately continue to voice. That's why I don't see Oliver's death as the herald of my own. When the weekly statistics are compiled and released, they give us an idea at once precise and abstract of our personal chances of dying, and we can always hope to be among those who slip through the fatal net. *The New York Times* recently assigned a survival average of eighteen months to patients stricken with pneumonia and twenty-four months to victims of Kaposi's sarcoma. I know AIDS victims whose illness began five years ago. Even the Fates tire in the end, as did the Nazi butchers, and a few souls are able to escape from the land of the dead.

Freud wondered if the impossibility of imagining one's own annihilation might be the source of the so-called heroic deeds of daredevils. In our case, it is our physical pain and the decision to take dangerous drugs that might be called heroic, rather than our daring to brave death. Since I haven't yet taken some of the precautions adopted by AIDS patients, such as writing a will, my behavior could be construed as thoughtlessness and crazy optimism. Or might it be superstition? When death rears its head, and neither fate nor the course of the virus may be predicted, superstition will creep in. They never lit three cigarettes on a match in trenches because the third light was supposed to draw the fatal bullet. Whenever I'm waiting for the results of my T4/T8 blood tests, I try to guess what they'll be, using evidence that bears no logical relation to the quality of my blood sample. People who live in a world of violence, where death is a constant and daily life is full of surprises—gangsters, for example—take superstition very seriously. Confronted with the super rationality of institutionalized medicine, we need an escape outlet of nonsense and tricks, the sorts of foolishness children spontaneously adopt for relief from their inexplicable anxieties. This is why I would never dare tell myself that I'm out of danger or that everything is going well. The very fact of saying such a thing out loud or in petto might tempt the enemy (the evil spirits, the *ma qwi* my Cambodian nurse would tell me about when I was a child) to lob over a shell especially meant to show me that the war has only just begun. I'm also afraid that others might think me naïvely overconfident.

This unnatural slaughter of young people makes everything relative. I'm convinced that certain AIDS patients, after enduring the loss of their best friends, somehow resent the elderly citizens back on the home front who have already enjoyed a long life but still fear illness and death, still complain about their little problems, wrapped up as they are in the senile egotism that often protects older people from the indifference they inspire in a society fixated on youth and health. And now we've prematurely caught up with them. In the ophthalmologist's waiting room, I was irritated by an exasperating old lady who didn't want to let the nurse give her a shot for her angioscopy. I've seen mere kids die without flinching while their mothers looked on, still smiling bravely, and I was completely unmoved by this old woman's childish stubbornness. I used to respect the elderly, but now I think they owe me some consideration precisely because they've been able to live so long. It's only since the virus recruited me into its ranks that I've become so aggravated by the insignificance of minor civilian dramas, which the more insensitive still dare to grumble about, the way I used to myself.

I can't stand it when civilians talk about AIDS. What do they know about it? How can they claim any authority when they're completely untouched by it, without a single wound or symptom? My only consolation is that they're terrified of catching it, of already harboring the disease. I'm being unfair, I know, because if healthy people didn't discuss AIDS, I'd secretly reproach them for their heartless indifference. I would simply like them to bow down before us, humbly accept our moods and caprices, and keep the relief effort running smoothly as a form of penance for their glowing good health. How can I resent them when I myself used Oliver's corpse as protection from enemy attacks, the quick saved by the dead? If AIDS comes to get me, I'll huddle down beneath my lover's body so I won't be found. That's why I play dead whenever the virus comes too close. I cancel all appointments and lie low until things take a turn for the better. People tell me: "You shouldn't stay shut in like that, a bit of air would do you good." But if I hide sheepishly at home, it's because the enemy is lying in wait for me just outside my front door: the germs of my fellow passengers on the subway, the piercing wind in late April, the changes in temperature, the food in restaurants are all so many torpedoes targeted in my direction. So I batten down the hatches and dive beneath the waves like a submarine, waiting for the enemy fleet to pass overhead, hoping that they won't find me on their radar screens. Like Anne Frank again, in her tiny room.

This absolute division between the two worlds

and their respective concerns is also a temporal barrier. Those who become ill must quickly forget who they are and everything they've been up until that moment. They must strip off their civilian personalities and habits in order to relearn how to live as soldiers. I have to erase all my peacetime reflexes, everything I know about good manners and savoir-vivre, all the things that gave me pleasure, and my deepest, innermost thoughts. To survive, you must die and be reborn in a new incarnation of your own making: aggressive, resolute, austere, and disciplined. Discipline is our only hope of survival, and it's the first lesson to be impressed upon people with AIDS. As a veteran of the student rebellion of '68, I've always hated discipline insofar as it meant the obligation to follow ridiculous orders issued by idiotic authorities. But one must temper one's soul so that it may withstand the strain of this life. I and all my generation grew up in a climate of national and international détente, a climate in which discipline seemed an old-fashioned and reactionary idea. That makes it all the more difficult to call upon the resources of discipline in the present crisis, but without it, our army would be lost. We are all struggling, the rest of society as well as my comrades and I, to resist the grim fascination exerted by this juggernaut.

PHOENIX

IT WAS THROUGH WRITING, that most solitary of acts, that I first sensed the true dimensions of our plight: an entire generation was floundering in the shadows of this sudden epidemic. I then convinced myself that by lighting a candle in the darkness I might help dispel a few of these oppressive shadows with the faint illumination cast by my diary. This torchlight parade would also allow us to stand up and be counted in our own lifetime instead of figuring only in obituaries.

Writing makes you less afraid, especially for yourself. In letters to your parents, you have to minimize the danger, reassure them, persuade them that they'll see you again and that everything they read in the papers is quite exaggerated. You can't dishearten civilians. If I were ever to let on that I'm afraid, everyone would panic, and the rush of pity would lower my immune defenses. The news in the letters I receive is all about family worries, financial difficulties, and especially minor health problems. It all seems so futile! Yet I realize that I once shared these concerns, and that if ever I make it back home again after the armistice, I'll return to the same old preoccupations, but with a new attitude this time. The serenity and health of others seem as though they would go on forever, and their pleasures are enhanced in my eyes by my misfortunes. Conversely, I can understand the terrible upheaval a serious illness brings into other people's lives. It's only now that I fully grasp the meaning of the words "She has cancer" and comprehend the true extent of the devastation thus visited on someone's life from that moment on. I would like those who can to enjoy their good health, and at the very least I would like my suffering to be useful, in a sense, by showing people how much they should treasure their relative happiness. The happiness of not being trapped in the living hell of Verdun.

Living in this hell is the only way to understand that the actual experience of something dreadful is sometimes easier to bear than what one has feared and imagined, or heard about in the media. It would be useless and hypocritical on my part to claim that AIDS is livable, but the rest of society's irrational terror might lead to the adoption of draconian measures, because they forget that we're still human beings, and the illness doesn't dispose of us as quickly as they may think. It's in everyone's interest to make something almost commonplace out of AIDS and its victims. To my great surprise, when I was diagnosed as having the virus I felt miraculously relieved. The great collapse I had dreaded for so long had at last occurred, had already occurred, in fact, and I hadn't even realized it! Only when Sonnabend detected the first traces of Kaposi's sarcoma in my intestines did I learn officially that I had nothing more to fear. I didn't need to hide out anymore: the cops had finally nabbed me.

I shortly discovered that I was sufficiently devoted to the defense of my personal liberties—including the supreme liberty, life itself—to take up arms without a qualm. I had been saying all along, "If I've got AIDS, I won't wait for the end. I'll commit suicide after blowing everything (including my health)." The day I was called up, however, there I was in my brand-new uniform, ready to lead the charge against pneumocystic carinii pneumonia. I had unwittingly prepared myself psychologically and physically for combat beforehand, like a reserve officer, throughout the entire period preceding my first opportunistic illness. I now understand that I unconsciously began my training the moment I learned that my test was positive and long before I became ill. It was disconcerting to be in the front line and at the same time reflect: "Well, today wasn't so bad," or "This week hasn't been all that terrible." Every day isn't catastrophic, and even bad news doesn't seem so worrisome once you've become something of a veteran. On the other hand, I've seen some youngsters treat the notice of positive test results as if it were a death warrant, when it's really only a declaration of war. Things are far from over at that point, and there's much that can be done, but because those untested recruits don't understand this yet, they have nervous breakdowns before they've even taken the train to the front.

Kristine tells me about her friend Joe, who is in the throes of youthful despair at the news that his lover has been sent into action and is now hospitalized, while he himself has just received his call-up notice in the form of a positive Elisa test. Dying so young is a bitter reality of war and AIDS: in both cases one must learn much sooner than one expected to come to grips with the idea of death. Once accidental or unlikely for those under sixty-five, death becomes a statistical inevitability with war and AIDS. Eric informs me that at a recent conference on the disease, Larry Kramer, one of the first AIDS militants, asked half his listeners to stand up, and then told them that they would be dead in five years. That was his way of making them realize no one is safe. Wars aren't won by soldiers sitting on their hands in a pillbox.

Once they begin showing the first signs of weakening in their immune systems, those young, well-muscled New Yorkers, so redolent of good health, become like recruits still full of energy in their spanking clean uniforms, but who might well be unrecognizable in six months. Like Fabrizio at Waterloo in Stendhal's novel, they don't yet understand anything about the soldiers, diseases, and researchers

maneuvering all around them. People whose AIDS
has just been confirmed should try to introduce a
certain rationality into the apparent chaos of this
epidemic and forget about the image they have of
previous AIDS patients, an image that is disturbing,
romantic, demonic, prematurely "otherworldly,"
and largely fostered by the media. AIDS remakes us
suddenly into adolescents for whom life is an
enigma: no adult has yet returned from this initia-
tion rite to help us pass the test.

I recently ran into this problem myself when Sonnabend asked me to telephone an AIDS patient coping with his first CMV infection and explain to him
what my own treatment was like, in the hope of
reassuring him—in vain, as it turned out. I talked
for over an hour with this man in his early thirties
whom fate had assigned to my platoon. Despite his
obvious intelligence and sensitivity, he hadn't yet
adopted the martial spirit that might have released
him from his terror. The expression he used most
frequently—"I dread"—seemed very revealing to
me. He was refusing to have the necessary tests per-
formed because they might be painful. I told him
that in so doing he was letting the enemy close in
on him without giving himself the means to determine the strength and tactics of the opposing forces.
I'm going to set out on a lecture tour to indoctrinate
the troops if this sort of thing keeps up.

If our prewar persona doesn't die away, we our-

selves die. We won't survive without the persever-
ance and strictness we scoffed at back when we were
healthy. One of the heroes in *All Quiet on the Western Front* remarks bitterly that in school he was never
taught the things he needed to know in wartime.
No one had told him, for example, that it's better
to thrust a bayonet into an enemy soldier's abdomen
than his rib cage because it's easier to pull the
weapon out. If we don't want to be wiped out, we
have to shed the cocoonlike attitude that some of
us favor. It's not enough to start off with a strong
ego and lots of ambition, because these attributes
can even prove to be obstacles. Those who refuse
to fling themselves flat on their bellies—in the mud,
if necessary—will be cut down by enemy surprise
attacks. Anyone who thinks first of his looks, the
charm and decorum of his previous lifestyle, or the
snappy crispness of his uniform is in danger of collapsing when his body itself comes under assault.
Narcissistic grounds must be ceded to the enemy in
the hope of saving essentials; there'll be time enough
later for figuring out how to disguise hair loss caused
by chemotherapy.

The maturer souls among us are more easily re-
signed to that gray area where I live, halfway between a healthy white and a deathly black. Younger
people, though, tend to see everything in black or
white, period. The loss of muscle tone, suppleness,

hair (so closely associated with virility) is the coup
de grâce for those egotists who refuse to change
their lives, give up being attractive, and accept the
alteration in their appearance. I'm ready to turn into
a toad if that will allow me to go on living. Being
able to obey an order instantly, without flinching,
can mean the difference between life and death.

One must learn to accept being scarred. The saber
cuts of Kaposi's sarcoma have left marks on many
a young and once seductive face, permanent marks
that no amount of makeup can ever erase. If only
these youths could derive a bit of glory from them
at least, like brave legionnaires, but the story they
have to tell is instead a sorry one. Woe to the van-
quished. That's the ultimate fate of people with
AIDS, to be losers in a society obsessed with winning. From the moment someone is stricken with
AIDS, all his previous accomplishments are retro
actively annulled. Cut down in their youth or middle
age, these people become entirely defined by their
deaths. When I watch the films of Rock Hudson
now, I see them in the light of his harrowing end.
These crises obliterate the past, disrupt the present,
and rewrite the future. A member of Congress has
just died of AIDS. He tried to make people believe
he was the victim of a contaminated blood trans-
fusion, but his secret homosexual past rapidly became public knowledge. His previous history, his

political career, the numerous progressive bills he had drafted, all this was forgotten in an instant. His AIDS overshadowed everything, thus depriving him of his past life retroactively and forever. When the soldier in *Paths of Glory* is executed by a firing squad, his former life is sullied in the same way and all his exploits effaced. A father killed in action remains a soldier in uniform to his children, just as they saw him on his last leave, even if he lived thirty-five years as a civilian and only six months at the front. Shame, even when unmerited, is as indelible as glory.

For the first time, a disease seems to be choosing its victims. In *Illness as Metaphor*, Susan Sontag contrasts tuberculosis with cancer. AIDS reconciles and combines the various aspects of these two diseases: it afflicts members of clearly defined communities, as does every contagious illness (cholera, plague), but also seems to select each victim for a precise and appropriate reason. In the same way, war threatens a given community (an ethnic group, soldiers, the inhabitants of a besieged city) while also picking and choosing among its victims, harvesting those who act irrationally or expose themselves to greater danger. Stories and films about war give death a dramatic and exemplary meaning when it strikes down a particular character, as if it were confirming this or that personality trait. There are groups at risk in war too. Death on the battlefield may sometimes redeem a coward or villain, just as a person with AIDS dies in such agony that his errors and sins (supposed or real) are burned away on the pyre of his fevers and suffocations.

I haven't been struck down yet, but I'm definitely an invalid, one whose wound is still more or less invisible, luckily. The peripheral catheters I carry inserted in my skin—and which I hide under bandages or long sleeves—are like the wooden legs or prostheses of disabled war veterans. In *The Best Years of Our Lives*, a film about GIs coming home in 1945, a crippled soldier tries to return to active civilian life, just as we AIDS patients attempt to keep our jobs and continue living a life as normal as possible, for as long as people let us. I have to beg my usual dentist to keep me on as a patient despite my AIDS and the fact that his assistants and receptionists are terrified by my visits. He might lose his clientele if they ever learned that I'd been drafted by the virus. Our social reintegration is compromised by rumors about the epidemic, something that disabled war vets are spared at least. If the people with whom I ride on the subway knew that I return every day from the AIDS front, they'd flee from me in panic. I'm as frightening as a gruesomely disfigured multiple amputee.

How could I forget the horror that I inspire in myself as well as in others? The Terror has invaded my daily life, even during its quieter moments, and I cannot watch television, read a newspaper, or just flip through a fashion magazine without seeing an advertisement for condoms, an obituary for someone famous struck down by AIDS, or a report on some new drug.

My first impulse, which turned out to be a good one, was to insist on living my life one day at a time. This means that each morning is the dawn of a new illness, the dice are constantly rethrown, and whatever has gone before is not decisive. There are some people who are doomed, once they've reached a given stage of weakness, because their bodies can no longer resist the virus. Things begin to happen fast, and the moment of surrender can even be predicted a few weeks in advance. On the other hand, fortunately, the thoughtless and sadistic death sentences handed down by certain doctors—and all the media—quite often turn out to be premature.

The unexpected moves the illness can make must be accepted as a diabolical game of chance. Our fear springs from our ignorance of the enemy's battle plans and intentions. Our spies—the blood tests of the immune system—are supposed to give us a glimpse of this hidden world, smuggling out top-secret coded information, but we still don't know how to decipher all the codes. The latest scientific discoveries don't allow us to anticipate everything that will happen, and so the doctor must keep a close eye on each development as it occurs. The illness is even more perplexing to the beginner, who goes crazy over an impressively high but fundamentally insignificant and short-lived fever, but neglects the insidious progress of his candidiasis infection, a subtle but sinister indication of the weakening of his immune defenses. That's what makes the disease exciting, this chess match between two adversaries. One of them is the blind creation of destructive natural forces, while the other, although initially clumsy and overawed by his opponent's massive strength, slowly becomes more sure of himself. We discover the chinks in the armor of AIDS as we go along.

So I wake up every day wondering about the quality of the bowel movements I'll have, which seem magically independent of my diet and the medicines I take. These daily skirmishes are more important and symbolic to me than an overview of the war seen as a whole. And yet the most concrete image of the disease raging in me isn't these bouts of diarrhea revealing the weakening of my intestines. Nor is it the dark spots of Kaposi's sarcoma on the mucosa of my bowels, which I saw thanks to a fiber-optics camera slipped like a periscope deep into my digestive tract, sending back exclusive pictures of this world of illness where enemy frigates threaten my beleaguered submarine. No, I was first truly seized with terror when I saw a film showing cells magnified millions of times being attacked in vitro by the HIV virus: the speed with which it invaded and captured the cell was chilling, much more so than my own symptoms. It haunts me still.

MEDUSA

BEHIND THE PROFOUND FEAR that grips a soldier in action lies more than artillery shells, bombers, and long-range missiles. It's a primitive fear, the fear of bodily harm and imminent death. In the same way, it's not so much this or that opportunistic illness that terrifies an AIDS patient, but the enemy lurking behind the façade of initials: it could be the NLF, the KKK, or the PLO, any organization whose aura of secrecy makes it seem all the more powerful and sinister. AIDS reinvents guerrilla warfare, since the traditional weapons of medicine are helpless before this subtle new form of aggression. True guerrilla tactics are similarly aimed at a country's immune defenses and centered on psychological warfare. Great conflicts have always included an element of propaganda, but AIDS is a fascinating and elusive foe that baffles traditional medicine by attacking where least expected. The slightest breakthrough or advance by the virus, the most innocuous rise in temperature, no matter how quickly jugulated, is perceived—especially in the beginning of the struggle—as a dramatic event illustrating how easily the enemy can capture vital territory. I feel like those commanders who know their situation is hopeless and resolve simply to kill as many of their attackers as possible before being overrun, preferring to die with their boots on rather than lower the flag. When one knows the enemy gives no quarter, what point is there in surrender except to cut short one's own suffering? In certain besieged cities, many inhabitants prefer to commit suicide by jumping from the ramparts to avoid witnessing the enemy's triumph. My former neighbor on Bank Street slit his wrists in his apartment the very evening he learned that his AIDS had become active.

We're all the more vulnerable to fear in that our mobilization by the virus too often leads to the loss of our jobs, even our homes if we live alone, or the breakup of our families if we're married. How many couples have been tested by one partner's case of AIDS? The other partner feels both guilty and frustrated. Should one continue to lead a normal life, or go into a kind of supportive isolation with the patient? Should one lavish constant encouragement on the invalid, or think of oneself while the other is in the hospital? Some people go half crazy and almost dread the return or the recovery of their partners, from whom they separate themselves mentally and emotionally at first, then physically and legally. Perhaps they can't bear the prospect of losing their lovers in spite of all their best efforts, and want to avoid the inevitable suffering and dramatic scenes. The patient in remission then realizes that his home has been devastated by separation and illness. It's asking a lot from people who are generally young and still healthy to expect them to remain faithful out of solidarity to companions more overwhelmed each passing day by the obligations and preoccupations thrust on them by their illness. Such a companion, once beloved, is no longer the same person, no longer himself. So why wait for the quite hypothetical return of this stranger, this unfamiliar AIDS patient? A GI's wife is sometimes too young to shut herself up in her apartment until her soldier returns, and she seethes with rage and frustration at wasting her best years in such a gloomy life. The lovers—especially the young ones—of AIDS patients become estranged from their partners in much the same way, not from fear of contagion (it would be too late, in any case), but because the illness compels them to deal with the forces of death, abnegation, and duty, while the forces of life within them clamor for the peacetime pleasures of the past. They don't want to deny themselves these pleasures by fighting for a cause that is not yet their own. Of course, there are also thousands of exemplary partners who care for their lovers until the last breath, writing to them whenever they're apart and making sure they have all the things they need when they're off in the trenches of a hospital ward.

When a patient is abandoned by his family and friends, organizations such as the Gay Men's Health

Crisis may help by assigning "buddies" to visit him, providing companionship and moral support to the lonely AIDS victim. Make no mistake: this disease puts human relationships to the test in a grueling and pitilessly revealing manner. The ordeal of AIDS brings out not only strengths and weaknesses of character in individuals but also the solidity or instability of relationships formed in time of health. Brought face to face with death and the sudden revelation of the essential workings of life, we have grown more mature. The intimate circle of friends and relations, the network of professional contacts, the everyday round of dealings with the electrician, the dentist, deliverymen—all are shattered when your AIDS becomes impossible to hide, as frightening and inescapable as a yellow Star of David. And one clings all the more to what remains of the normal life one led before the virus struck.

Many people with AIDS, although still able to work, are forced out of their jobs or leave them voluntarily. They can manage to get by, one hopes, thanks to disability pensions, and some of them retreat into a kind of limbo, giving up their careers, running the danger of opting out of life as they become more dependent on the illness itself. Dishonorably discharged from life, so to speak, they retire ingloriously from the field at such an early age that they must somehow feel guilty at becoming a burden to society. I work only part-time now, which means that I find myself rather on the sidelines in my professional milieu. This special schedule could be psychologically dangerous for me, since it loosens my hold on everyday life, but shouldn't I also pay attention to my body's need for rest?

An AIDS patient who no longer works quickly panics if he winds up alone in a hospital room or, even more frightening, abandoned in his apartment by people he once thought were his friends. That's when he contemplates a cherished portrait, rereads a letter from home for the umpteenth time, and dreams, not necessarily of victory, but of an end to the fighting, a truce. The mental alienation of the illness and the ominous silence all around him weigh heavily on his nerves. An AIDS patient on his own— someone whose partner is hospitalized, or already dead, or even just off at work—is lost in a stifling no-man's-land. The futile babble of TV and radio is powerless against the anguish, the oppressive sense of danger he feels. Illness thus has its own particular loneliness, even in the midst of an epidemic. Others may share your worries, but there comes a moment, after they've gone home, when you must return to the front alone. No one else can take your place if you wander into the path of an enemy bullet, that chance encounter with necessity provoked by war; men must be killed, and it so happens that in such and such a time and place, you make a perfectly acceptable corpse.

I never feel my solitude so keenly as when I watch passersby in the street from my window. The bomb fell on my house, not theirs. Now that I have AIDS, I'm more alone than I ever was in my entire life. It's a chill that the touching solicitude of my friends and relations can never dispel: they pile on the blankets of their warm affection, but I can't stop shivering. In an attempt to forget their distress, deaden their feelings, and bask in a bit of artificial warmth, some of my friends with ARC/AIDS turn to alcohol, tranquilizers, or illegal drugs. American soldiers in Vietnam tried to escape into these same artificial dreamworlds. I'd be afraid those useless remedies would overtax my strength, making me an easy target for the incorruptible virus.

Like those malingerers who surface in every army in the world, my twenty-five-year-old neighbor dying of AIDS has chosen a different way out: madness, a gentle madness, the simplest refuge from the other illness. The only difference is that he's not faking at all: he doesn't recognize anyone anymore, neither his doctors nor even his relatives. In his own way, he has cured himself. Unfortunately, he hasn't been evacuated, just interned in a hospital where he must breathe through tubes to counteract the collapse of his lungs. He's the living example of what loneliness and fear can do to fragile and inexperienced young people. My friend's delirium might well be caused by the effects of the virus on his brain, but in his case, signs of mental imbalance appeared quite rapidly in the course of his illness. This mass psychosis of the besieged afflicts us all to varying degrees. It can have a physical aspect, which may well be the cause of the chronic slight fevers often associated with lymphadenopathy and the early stages of the disease. This febrile state is just as much psychological as it is physical, and it leads AIDS patients to dash off in all directions, believe in all sorts of miracles, listen to all manner of quacks, pledge their souls to the Virgin or macrobiotics, and stock up on every kind of vitamin imaginable.

The interminable moves from one post to another and the long, uneventful marches sometimes give rise to a general feeling of boredom in the barracks. The main activity becomes simply killing time, which is exactly what we're running out of in the long haul. Since the pleasures and distractions of the mind are still permitted, the intellectuals among us are envied by other AIDS patients, who find themselves disconcerted by the sudden emptiness of their days. Sartre's account of his mobilization during the "phony war" (1939–40) comes to mind. His constant reading kept up his morale and saved him from the gloomy moods that beset his bunkmates. Now that most of our peacetime diversions—sports, cruising, going out on the town—are off-limits, we have to find ways of amusing ourselves in the evening, but also during the day if we're no longer working, we who have taken sabbatical leave of life. Ever since I began keeping this diary, time has become dear to me again. The great paradox of this disease is that it devalues time just when the approach of death renders time so very precious. Both the most lucid and the most desperate AIDS patients behave in the same way, for opposite reasons: they cling to the habits that structure their days and pretend that their peacetime existence has never been disrupted. We need to reinvent our lives, to find a rhythm adapted to our new circumstances, but this endeavor is beyond the strength of many of us, even those who used to find their former daily routines burdensome but now look back on them with nostalgia.

Boredom is a more subtle enemy than fear. To break up the monotony of hospital schedules and the routines we must follow at home, the more courageous or extroverted among us become AIDS militants, organizing a collective movement and creating, for the first time in history, a self-governed union of patients. Those who are more creative also try to entertain us while keeping our spirits up. In San Francisco they've put together a kind of USO theater (called "The AIDS Show") specifically aimed at AIDS patients. This collection of songs and sketches is meant to draw the audience into the performance, in the hope that they can forget their despair for a moment and even laugh about it, the

way one makes fun of the enemy or a stupid ser-
geant, cutting them down to size. The cares and
terrors of a life with AIDS are exorcised in these
good-natured comedy routines, which give the patients a sense of solidarity—a bit artificial, perhaps,
but reassuring. One almost feels like singing along,
joining in with something in the spirit of 1942: *Boogie
Woogie Man, This Number Is for Uncle Sam*, or Alice
Faye's torch song, *No Love, No Nothing, Not 'Til My
Baby Comes Home*. Touring the hospitals, "The
AIDS Show" is put on before an audience of am-
bulatory patients in the front line, and it gives them
the courage to continue, showing them that the rest
of the world (or part of it, at least) cares about their
struggle.

Although I can clearly see the universal dimensions of our campaign, I don't dare join the militants'
Resistance. I'm content to listen to their Free French
broadcasts by reading the magazines they publish
and following accounts of their exploits in the press.
Like Sartre and Simone de Beauvoir during the Oc-
cupation, I don't feel the call to become a "terrorist."
It's not something I feel I'm capable of doing. Instead, I do my part by writing this diary-tract and
signing my petition.

What I find most difficult is distinguishing between reality and fabrication when crises stir up their
inevitable confusion. Rumor has become a form of
communication well suited to this present period of

official mendacity. In fact, we are long-winded producers and greedy consumers of reports that spread all the faster for their patent absurdity. When it first appeared on the scene, AIDS was as mysterious as a punishment from heaven, so rumors flew thick and fast. One of them involved germ warfare, and its persistence reflects the spirit of general paranoia this epidemic inspires in groups at risk. Some say the virus was deliberately isolated and cultivated in CIA laboratories, and those who claim to be in the know maintain that it was part of a plan to bring Cuba to its knees once and for all. According to this science-fiction scenario, an accident in which a test tube spilled its contents into an open wound supposedly unleashed the epidemic now ravaging the planet. An even more paranoid contingent insists that the CIA set out to eliminate American deviants, homosexuals and drug addicts, intending to study the evolution of the disease in situ and in vivo before using it abroad. In this version of "The Sorcerer's Apprentice," AIDS went out of control, spreading first throughout the Western nations because of their more liberal morals. The current epidemic would thus be the complete reverse of its original conception, which was to be an attack on Communism. The idea that the AIDS epidemic was deliberately plotted by a small group of mysterious conspirators has no appeal for me; I see the epidemic as the tragic result of an unfortunate chain of circumstances.

In time of war or a similar emergency, self-destructive tendencies are suddenly stirred up by feelings of even hypothetical inferiority. Anyone who admits to a moral flaw might very well suffer from a physical one. A heterosexual man does not generally introduce anything into his own body, so he risks nothing and doesn't give an adversary any opening, unlike a homosexual, who greedily ingests, absorbs, allows a foreign organ to burrow inside him, welcomes it with open arms into the most intimate citadels of his body. The armed men of this Trojan horse are not only the sperm cells but also the many viruses that secretly enter the blood of Troy, a consenting and careless prey, bent on its own destruction. The oppression of the American homosexual community by the puritan majority had diminished somewhat over the past twenty years, and like the Trojans, overjoyed at what we thought to be the departure of the Greeks, we slowly let down our guard. But the sexual revolution (and the spread of drug addiction) was only a ruse. The soldiers were hidden in the womb of the horse, in the needle, in the phallus. No sooner had the homophobes lifted their siege than the massacre began. The Trojan War, Western culture's archetype of the fated inevitability of armed conflict, is also the original, primordial war of our civilization. Giraudoux, in *Tiger at the Gates*, and Sartre, in *The Flies*, have portrayed the inescapable workings of the mechanism that sparks the conflict, despite the best intentions of some among the future adversaries. My AIDS was equally unavoidable. The pathological process thrown into gear inside me without my knowledge, at a time when the existence of the virus was as yet unknown, is marked with the sign of fate. The illness was bound to declare itself, though I tried by all possible means to avoid that explosion of the death instinct once its origins had become clear. My AIDS and the Trojan War were brought about by Love, by Aphrodite, the patron deity of Troy, goddess of sexuality and even lust. It was through her patronage, through the sexual flame she ignited in Paris and Helen, that Troy was symbolically lost. The sensual abandon and derangement induced by the seductive Aphrodite led directly to the blindness of Priam and his men, who decided to bring the wooden horse within the walls of the city despite Cassandra's warnings. It says in the *Odyssey* that the Trojans tried four times before they managed to bring in the horse, which was too large for the gates of their city. Six years ago, American Cassandras were accused by the majority of Trojans, myself among them, of playing into the enemy's hands by calling for a halt to all erotic revels until the AIDS horse had revealed what was concealed in its belly. At a time when the first few hundred victims had already fallen, most drug addicts and homosexuals suspected the authorities of trying to interfere with their personal liberties by concocting a new disease out of thin air.

The bombed-out ruins of this war aren't just our skeletal bodies, gnawed by worms and parasites, those insatiable vultures, but are also the domain of gay sexuality. The homosexual city has been pillaged by the invaders. One by one, our fortresses—the baths, the sex clubs, even the gay bars and our thickets in the parks—have fallen beneath the double onslaught of puritanism and AIDS, while those who regularly frequented those now unhealthy places soon found themselves on the front line. The entire American gay community has been forced to retreat by the revived hostility of a society terrified of AIDS. Our militants are obliged to defend the positions we've already won, in an attempt to keep the virus from wiping out all the hard-won rights of homosexuals in the Western world, or at the very least, to limit its devastating effect on our liberties.

Fritz Zorn, the author of *Mars*, kept the diary of his illness from cancer like a disillusioned pacifist. The war he lost is not my war. I don't recognize myself in his petulant struggles or his defeatist acceptance of disease. "I've lost the war, a war against whom, in fact? Hard to say, although I've got plenty of words at hand: my parents, my family, the surroundings in which I grew up, bourgeois society, Switzerland, the system. A bit of all that is included in what I'll call the principle that is hostile to me. . . . I am now in the concentration camp being gassed by my share of parental heritage." The author of those lines is dead now, but many people with AIDS might be tempted to think as he does, at least unconsciously. They accuse others of having provoked the opening of hostilities, and they refuse to take part in the war. Other AIDS patients who haven't the exhibitionistic tendencies of Zorn or myself confront the enemy in silence, all the more courageously in that this combat doesn't excite them as it does me. In my moments of doubt, I see myself as the braggart Falstaff, aflame with resolve as long as the enemy is out of earshot, but humble and crestfallen whenever AIDS draws near.

It's true that the disease provides fertile ground for the most outrageous misconceptions, which has led everyone to lose their grip on common sense. AIDS patients are often confused by their suffering and their obsession with the virus, but public authorities can't hide behind that excuse to justify the waste of time and effort during the first few years of the epidemic. Throwing all scientific precision to the wind, the establishment fell back on explanations that were tautological or irrational, blaming factors such as certain lifestyles or the consumption of this or that drug. Paranoia drove some gay journalists to warn their readers against eating pork, thus implying that all cases of AIDS were actually some kind of "swine flu." Their reaction reminded me of those Frenchmen who rebaptized the Germans as "krauts," thinking they were thereby making a contribution to the war effort. Just as spy fever made everyone mistrust those with German names, certain people, places, and products are now judged to be dangerous without any proof whatsoever and solely on the basis of rumor. Substances like vitamin C, penicillin, and various mysterious liquids are suddenly touted in a manner as arbitrary as it is peremptory. The general public no longer puts any faith in the statements and reassurances of doctors either. The heterosexual population, which is not well informed on the subject, is of course ready to believe the wildest nonsense, but there are also healthy homosexuals who haven't been called up for duty yet who break off all contact with former friends or lovers who have contracted AIDS. My nurse told me he had to cut the hair of one of his patients himself because the sick man's friends— some of whom are hairdressers—had refused to do him this favor. In such cases the AIDS patient is like a spy infiltrating society. Paranoia, which always flourishes during wars and epidemics, creates a climate of suspicion: a strange accent, an effeminate waiter, and everyone starts worrying. In the eyes of heterosexual society, homosexuals have become the enemy within, a fifth column of the third sex.

The disproof of an alarmist rumor doesn't prevent those who started it from launching another one just as absurd, since people with AIDS are as credulous as the inhabitants of a country at war. Deprived of hope, they're ready to grasp at any chance of a miraculous solution, believing the worst all the while. It's because of this kind of idle talk that certain homosexuals shun their former haunts, which they now equate with recruitment centers for AIDS.

Some of the clandestine rumors going around are unfortunately confirmed by obituary notices. Public opinion manages to elude protective censorship and find out which celebrities are stricken with the virus, the fallen angels of AIDS. Some of them try at first to deny their defeat, their AIDS, their homosexuality, or they confess the truth at the last minute, like Rock Hudson. Still others are finally unmasked after their death, like Liberace or Perry Ellis. The well-intentioned lamentations of the press over the heavy toll AIDS has taken among artists strike me as indecent. World War I wasn't horrible simply because it cut short the lives of writers like Apollinaire and Rupert Brooke. It's condescending to single out gay artists and court jesters from the mass of AIDS victims in this artificial manner. Journalists seem more interested in the entertainment these late celebrities once provided the general public than in the fate of human beings destroyed by the epidemic. But it is true that the loss of all these creative individuals represents a major defeat for life, proving that even those in the best position to defend themselves, those able to afford the finest medical advice and treatments, are mowed down by AIDS like the French at Dien Bien Phu. Wartime censorship may perhaps delay or forbid the spread of bad news, just as the Nazis tried to hide from Germany the fact that von Paulus had surrendered at Stalingrad, but sooner or later the fall of our fortresses makes the headlines.

It's hard to understand how AIDS can be an occult phenomenon, the subject of superstitious rumors, and at the same time provide a huge televised spectacle, rich in exciting new developments. AIDS puts us through our death agonies in the glare of the public eye, yet makes us feel forgotten and abandoned by everyone. Thanks to technological progress, AIDS is the first deadly epidemic with live coverage, just as the war in Vietnam was the first televised war. AIDS has become an electronic event perceived as unreal even though it traumatizes the households into which it penetrates via the TV screen, thereby traumatizing the conscience of the entire nation. Voltaire said that war was a dreadful disease. AIDS is a dreadful war, waged outside the bounds of the Geneva Convention, but so picturesque, so fascinating, worth its weight in gold! The camera invariably seeks out the "victims" of the most spectacular battles. Its instinct for the sensational leads it to prefer the bald and wasted AIDS patient with the feverish, haggard look, lying in his hospital bed (preferably with a few tubes up his nose), to his companion who is still able to take care of himself and speak articulately about his condition. The camera solemnly closes in on the withered bodies, feeding greedily on the wounds of these men now incapable of uttering more than a few monosyllables, while the medical specialists, the generals, are interviewed at great length. We're so interesting to look at, lying silently on our stretchers. During the war in Vietnam, American television lingered pitilessly over the gravely wounded soldiers being unloaded from troop transports in Hawaii or California. The men didn't have to say anything; they had only to illustrate the disasters of war. Is not a stalwart silence the supreme virtue demanded of a soldier? Everyone knows it's best not to give us a chance at the microphone and that pictures deceive even better than words.

I agreed to allow a Dutch television crew to film in my apartment during one of my nurse's regular biweekly visits, and their presence imparted the aura of a religious service to the routine operations Dan and I perform. The phallic eye of the camera inevitably fixed itself on my distended vein, bulging below the tourniquet, then scrutinized my face, like an animal innocently and obscenely curious about my reaction. The cameraman, carrying his machine around on his shoulder, reminded me of the centaurs who were thought to possess ancient skills in medicine and magic. Once our collective voyeurism had been satisfied, the interviewer then asked me the two ritual questions always put to AIDS patients: "Do you feel lonely, and how has your life been changed?" My wife for ten years, Kristine, who is now my companion, was asked (in my absence): "How do you feel, watching him die before your very eyes?" She answered like a soldier, replying that I'm not dying of AIDS, but living with it, and that she is there to help me live with it. The entry of this camera and these strangers into my hermit's grotto drains some of the reality out of my illness; all at once my AIDS is projected onto the walls of my cave, and I don't recognize myself in this terrifying and deformed shadow that will appear on Dutch television. After the departure of these Red Cross observers who had come to inspect my camp, my loneliness returns with crushing force. All my life has been leading up to this, to AIDS, and I didn't realize it! Seen in this light, the satisfaction I felt at leaving a tangible record of my struggle, in these pages and on the videocassette, suddenly seems ridiculous. I'm not the first human being to suffer misfortune.

We've now finally understood that no one ever really wanted to find out what we thought about AIDS. The liberal doves, who support educating the public, and the reactionary hawks, who favor imposing discriminatory measures, debate loudly while we stand by. They fight to see who will take the helm, leaving us to drift in the confused current of opinion. I wish we could regain control—through mutiny, if necessary—of this Ship of Fools, tossed by the stormy seas of society's antiquated ideas and prejudices.

COMRADES IN AIDS

NOW MORE THAN EVER we must refuse to disown our native land, adopted though it may be; we must refuse to betray our friends. If the Afghans can fight fiercely to defend the desert they call home, then we ought also to fight for our beleaguered land, our homosexuality. Conditions there are now made even more difficult by AIDS, but the homosexual homeland has never been a place of milk and honey. The Falklands come to mind instead, rugged islands whose inhabitants are so attached to those few acres of snow and ice that they are willing to die in their defense. I don't see why we couldn't likewise cherish the country of our choice without having to apologize to strangers for our devotion to such a rocky and infertile place.

On the other hand, the dichotomous image I once had of the world and the unconscious distinctions I used to make between my straight and gay friends have faded away. No longer living as one or the other, castrated by illness, I find myself freed from the blinkers formerly imposed on me by the conformist pressures of my own minority group. Those sexual blinkers have been replaced—quite involuntarily—by those of illness. The dividing line between *us* and *them* no longer follows the boundary I created in the past. Everything is in ruins in this sexual no-man's-land where I now bivouac, and it's hard for me to remember what I'm fighting for.

During World War II, Hollywood produced many films which were not necessarily war movies but which celebrated the American myth, the élan of its generosity, sincerity, and enjoyment of life. The last "good" war against totalitarianism. This affirmation of life and shared values is strangely absent from the world of people with AIDS. Life has already withdrawn from our gatherings, where we recite the monotonous litany of deaths and bemoan our current misfortunes like old ladies chatting together after Mass. We must constantly shake off these defeatist tendencies, this apathy that paralyzes us even quicker than the virus does. What we need are art forms that might symbolize our sacred Union, allowing us to identify with our struggle. We don't have any of those martial hymns that boost morale with a feigned unanimity of spirit while drowning out the sound of cannon fire and the shouts of protestors. In my case, the culture of illness has driven out the culture of deviance and homosexuality.

At the very moment when he has most need of stability, the homosexual suffering from AIDS often feels driven by his illness to disown what he is, his raison d'être, thereby loosening his ties to the gay community. Didn't I resolve to renounce that sexuality which once defined me so completely, in order to fight with all my strength? Like the Algerians or the Vietnamese, whose courage and determination were reinforced by their strong feelings of national community, we ought to find our way back somehow to the ancient camaraderie of our sex, an oasis in this desert of gloom and confusion that confronts us now.

I'm not the only one who feels helpless. The Trojan horse of AIDS brings out the weaknesses, hypochondria, homophobia, and egotism already gnawing away at those countries invaded by the virus. Reeling from the blow, our societies are tempted to grope blindly for the quickest, easiest solutions, just as some people turn to the army at the slightest sign of danger. Like Pétain before him, Reagan has chosen to ignore the conflict engulfing his country. I have watched in disbelief as the United States has shunted AIDS into the domain of the private sector. The government has "conducted" this disease in typical Reagan fashion, just like the Contra war in Nicaragua, by discreetly slipping it into the hands of private organizations. The authorities are counting on individual initiative and the invisible hand of the free market to save the day, restricting their own intervention to the minimum by simply coordinating these individual programs, and thereby contributing to the sense of isolation of forty thousand American AIDS victims abandoned to their own resources and public charity, because there's no longer any question of justice for all. A private company thus holds the power of life or death over those who seek to buy from it—at exorbitant prices—the only drug approved so far by the FDA for the treatment of AIDS: azidothymidine, or AZT. Why not carry the logic of this system to its obvious conclusion by organizing an auction of these grenades of hope, which each buyer would then carry off to his own little corner before pulling the pin?

It's such a dirty war that the task of coping with it is assigned to private contractors and militias, who can decide our fate, dead or alive. Our corpses are hastily cremated or buried by recalcitrant personnel who tack supplemental charges onto their bills to cover what they claim are necessary precautionary measures. Some won't come near us without gloves on even while we're alive—society's latest humiliating and sadistic little touch. I experience the uprooting of the AIDS community, its sudden social ostracism, in much the same way as Americans of Japanese descent in California lived through their internment in camps from 1941 to 1943. Their only crime was to be suspected of hampering the war effort, a suspicion based solely on the fact that they belonged to a group "at risk." So it's not too surprising that the idea of confining AIDS victims in camps surfaced in California in 1986. As for the Ba-

varian authorities and William Buckley, they've
come up with the idea of tattoos (would they be
the ritual decorations of brave warriors or the con-
venient identification numbers of concentration
camp prisoners?). Locking us up, a tactic favored
by those in France who remember the pogroms with
nostalgia, would effectively place us hors de combat
in death traps draped with the white flag of defeat
and unconditional surrender.

Discrimination is now legalized in the name of
hygiene. In wartime, soldiers are haunted by the
prospect of typhus, since even corpses can spread
the infection. The Germans hid behind this pretext
in 1941 when they built a wall around the Warsaw
Ghetto. They used typhus as a shield to mask discreetly their extermination of the Jews, a people who
have been accused since the Middle Ages of being
natural carriers of the disease. This time-honored
reflex terrifies the AIDS victims of today. Each new
incident reported in the press feeds our paranoia.
Now they're accusing us too of poisoning the wells
of Western societies—the sexual wells, in this case.

Some people are surprised that AIDS patients
have organized themselves into protective associa-
tions. People who suffer from tuberculosis, cancer,
and other diseases come together only through the
most contingent circumstances, quite outside their
own volition, and they feel only a superficial sense
of solidarity with other patients who share their

illness. We, on the other hand, have a real need for the kinds of support structures other patients readily find in society and in their professions and family relationships. These networks are infinitely more precarious for many homosexuals who have only recently arrived in the larger cities, far from their homes and families, and whose relatives may often be completely ignorant of their sexual orientation. Deprived of the normal channels of assistance used by heterosexuals when they are ill, AIDS patients—drug addicts or homosexuals—won't receive the consideration usually shown to the sick, nor can they count on the sympathy of the authorities. Quite on the contrary, they must cope in addition with the prejudices of their own society, which accuses them of fomenting disorder when they seek merely to defend themselves or even just to survive. Certain self-righteous individuals reproached the few Jews who resisted the Nazi police with the same crime of stirring up unrest and not going quietly into quarantine. In the land of health, the AIDS patient is in enemy territory, and becomes a stranger even to his colleagues, friends, and family.

Our new spirit of solidarity is the unexpected outcome of the paranoia haunting us all. Susan Sontag criticizes the paranoia lying behind the warlike images used by the press to describe the fight against cancer. Well, our AIDS is made of pure paranoia. I see in my figure of the Trojan horse a represen-

MORTAL EMBRACE : 131

tation of the psychosis already rampant in the gay
community before the epidemic, a psychosis that
has become the dominant characteristic of our own
perception of the illness on the individual and collective levels. In this diary, where everything stems
from my interpretations, everything is paranoid.
What I'm trying to do here is probe the depths of
my reality and draw my own conclusions, which are
vital to me even if others may find them absurd. In
"realist" war literature (*Les Croix de bois, All Quiet
on the Western Front, The Naked and the Dead*), the
protagonists are similarly wary of everyone else, of
the enemy, of civilians, but also of headquarters; no
one trusts anyone, and the most cynical viewpoints
find the readiest acceptance. Fighting under such
horrible conditions, one winds up hating even those
who are officially allies. AIDS patients are thus naturally suspicious, certainly lucid, but also extraor-
dinarily skeptical. Once embarked on this course of
doubt, they find it must remain the only course open
to them, and they systematically wage their own
personal war against the rest of the world, a world
untroubled by sickness. Of course, I can circulate in
an intolerant society thanks to the camouflage of
good health I take pains to wear at all times, but by
keeping ourselves invisible for as long as we can, we
confirm the preconceived ideas of the non-AIDS
world, which thus sees only those of us who are
already half dead and can't fight for their rights as

workers and citizens. When the police in the nation's capital put on plastic gloves before arresting lesbian demonstrators, can I be wrong in thinking that for much of the population we have become beings as frightening as zombies in a horror film, creatures that many wouldn't hesitate to strike down, as in *The Night of the Living Dead*, having once persuaded themselves that we were monsters with empty eyes, despite our human appearance, and intent on dragging them down with us into the abyss?

And so we're forced to fall back on a solidarity that strengthens our previous ties as members of an oppressed tribe, practitioners of ancestral rites. Like draftees from the same hometown or social milieu, we immediately feel drawn together by our affinities, by our common language. Jean-Pierre telephoned me yesterday from Paris to tell me that he has just been called up for duty and to ask for tips on the various treatments available in America for Kaposi's sarcoma. The international phone connection was a bad one, and I had the fleeting impression that we were exchanging restrained messages of commiseration and encouragement on field telephones left over from the Great War. What we are instinctively re-creating is a new Resistance network. We were already past masters at secrecy and dissimulation, which used to afford me great pleasure whenever I had occasion to exchange a look of complicity with one of my "fellows" in the heart of straight society, which remained oblivious to our intrigues.

In my daily life from now on, no one must suspect me of carrying so many explosives in my organic luggage. My pallor must not betray me. For a year I hid the fact that I had AIDS from my father as naturally as young men in the Resistance kept their activities a secret from their families so as not to worry them. Of course, their families suspected something, but they preferred being left in the dark. Belonging to a group exposed to danger gives us an ambiguous feeling of superiority, a sense of pride at having survived the rigors of AIDS so far, of having learned how to live with it. In the film *The Young Lions*, a woman says to one of the men on leave, "You soldiers, you always seem to think you belong to a superior race." The passwords used by AIDS patients (KS, PCP, CMV, T4/T8) create a sort of secret society within the gay community, an elite corps that demands respect from their peers, from those for whom, in a way, they have taken up arms. A new secret fraternity of signs, a freemasonry of codes, which sometimes unites us even with our doctors.

For obvious reasons, our first concern has been to protect our identities. Resistance fighters can't have their names and addresses flashed on a computer screen. So we use aliases when we are tested for the virus, since we don't trust any of the institutions that make those mealy-mouthed promises about keeping all AIDS data confidential. Next we become adept at arms trafficking, and channels have been set up to funnel smuggled Mexican, Canadian, or Israeli drugs into New York. In order to qualify for treatment with AZT, I had to have papers forged to certify a posteriori that a bronchoscopy had confirmed the presence of pneumocystic carinii pneumonia in my lungs. We're also forced to challenge the medical establishment itself, those collaborationists who treat with the enemy in an attempt to gain time. Resistance fighters don't want to gain just a few months, they want to liberate their country. By any means, legal or not, and even by acts of terrorism: radical gay groups like Act Up recently staged dramatic protests on Wall Street and in Washington against excessive profits earned by medical laboratories and the ban in the United States on drugs already approved for use in other countries. By treating us like guinea pigs, those in charge of research programs are abdicating their present responsibilities for an uncertain future. Doctors in the guerrilla movement, who tend to regard the FDA and other official institutions as the equivalent of the CIA, do everything they can to promote and finance illegal drugs and treatments, somewhat like American radicals who send money to the Nicaraguan government for their war against the Contras.

Until last year, there was a black market in New York for two drugs that hadn't yet received official approval from the all-powerful FDA, Ribavirin and AZT, and this is still the case for other experimental substances such as AL 721. Speculators sell our munitions as contraband. Isn't this the way guerrilla movements all over the world equip themselves? All's fair in love and war. If a certain drug can't be obtained legally, no one with AIDS would hesitate for a moment to make it himself, in the bathtub if necessary. AL 721, an Israeli discovery, is made on the sly by militants and distributed clandestinely at a church in my neighborhood. Terrorists sometimes blow themselves up with their homemade bombs, and I've no doubt that a few overzealous AIDS patients have burned themselves or shortened their own lives by making mistakes with chemical products believed to stimulate the immune system. The time has come when commandos without access to official ammunition depots must fend for themselves. I've spent my savings on a veritable arsenal of drugs stashed in my refrigerator, my war chest. Doctors warn us periodically against the dangers of overmedication threatening AIDS patients too eager to act for the sake of action.

Because of the particular risks I run, I make it my business to improvise a strategy rather freely inspired by the general battle plan of the authorities, who aren't always aware of what we're doing with our drugs. Like all pioneers, I have established an almost personal relationship with the enemy that obsesses me. In short, we respect each other, and I even feel a certain admiration for my adversary, which I mention here somewhat reluctantly for fear of seeming like a madman or a traitor. Of course the authorities, looking down on us through binoculars from their lofty heights, can observe and discern troop movements as yet invisible to me. There's no real difference between the behavior of a guerrilla and that of a rebellious patient. Exasperated by headquarters' timidity and indecisiveness, our soldiers sometimes resort to outright mutiny: lying to those responsible for medical protocols, taking drugs incompatible with the doctors' research, even throwing away the prescribed medicines.

Whenever I take a new experimental drug—and people fight desperately to be among those privileged to risk their lives—I feel as though I belong to a unit of shock troops parachuted behind enemy lines: already written off as a casualty, I'm entrusted with the task of spearheading the advance. Thanks to our reconnaissance missions, those who come after us will have a better idea of the immediate and long-term secondary effects of these drugs. I see myself slipping cautiously through the jungle of symptoms, followed at a distance by my doctor, who gives me my instructions over the phone after studying the results of my biweekly tests. Obliged to fa-

miliarize themselves with the topography of the
terrain, people with AIDS are prodigious readers of
information brochures, scientific articles, medical
journals, and the like, because they must become
proficient with their weapons so as not to be caught
short at a decisive moment. I know that if I begin
having difficulty breathing, I must immediately have
a blood test and a bronchoscopy to determine if the
problem is PC pneumonia, in which case large doses
of Bactrim are in order. Then I can only hope that
the enemy will back down in the face of such en-
lightened determination.

Victory belongs to those who outreason and out-
fox the enemy. Patience is an essential virtue in any
war of attrition. Instead of boasting and swaggering
around, one must devote oneself entirely to the com-
plicated and laborious job of undermining, day after
day, the actions of the invading virus, like the Vietcong digging their labyrinth of tunnels under the
very feet of their adversaries. Throughout the period
when I was only a healthy carrier of AIDS, I began
to prepare myself for the coming battle. Thus I was
able to build the landing strips vital to future operations, dig my immunological trenches, and
strengthen my resistance with long psychological
workouts. When the virus launched its first attack,
I was ready.

We're true freedom fighters, all of us, struggling
for our homosexual homeland.

FAREWELL TO AIDS

DISEASES, LIKE WARS, are difficult in the telling; those actually immersed in the struggle cannot communicate what they feel, especially in the beginning, when they lack all perspective on what is happening to them—and the others don't know what they're talking about. I'm not composing my war memoirs like a de Gaulle or a Churchill because I'm only a foot soldier, without any overall picture of the conflict. I'll tell my war stories to the young gays who come along after the miracle cure has been discovered, after the armistice has been signed. They'll shudder with horror at my senile reminiscences, but only for a moment; soon they'll return to their round of pleasures and forget this grim period in our collective history. Is anyone still interested in hearing about the Korean War? Anyway, a war cannot be recounted day by day. Only the outstanding events, the great, symbolic highlights—either individual or collective—are worthy of interest. Language is too rudimentary or too lazy to render adequately the slow parade of hours and days.

Like all forms of committed art, of *littérature engagée*, this book risks leaving its readers with a sense of frustration. My sieve of words inevitably dilutes the overpowering force of the AIDS phenomenon, merely retaining its cruder elements, since only the poetic vision of a William Blake could do justice to the myriad subtleties that truly define the impressionistic state of mind of someone with AIDS. And yet the awkwardness of a simple soldier pouring out his thoughts can be a point in his favor, since the immediacy of his experience helps make up for any lack of literary skill.

My unconscious hope is that this book, sprung from my brain like a cancerous growth, will become a monstrous appendage easily excised from my body. I fantasize that each phrase, each metaphor will stand in for one of my lymphocytes claimed by AIDS. In my world turned upside down, writing is not only a form of therapy but also a magical exercise. By confronting the epidemic through its reflection in my diary, I can hope to decapitate the Gorgon before it turns me to stone. The philter into which I thus plunge my anguish and obsession will become all the more effective as my audience grows. Each of my readers will become a soldier in my legion. I dream of indoctrinating and enlisting all those who read my words, so that they might save me. Once the umbilical cord between me and my book has been cut, I will perhaps find relief from my AIDS through this verbal exorcism, these words I strive to arrange in the proper order so that they will somehow weave the thread of logic indispensable to all ritual formulas of healing. These incantations are pronounced to achieve victory, to conjure up the spirits of those who have gone before me, the spirits of my homosexual ancestors, of those already sacrificed to AIDS, of the Great Sachem of gays, so that they may inspire me with a war chant and help me to dip my sword in the AIDS dragon's blood. Unfortunate Siegfried.

All's quiet on the front line; one can even hear birds singing, and a few buds have begun to swell not far from the barbed wire. A moment's peace, and we're able to forget the war. Then suddenly the bucolic landscape is torn apart by a murderous bombardment, and I wind up in the hospital after a week of relentless shelling. Death is ever near, ever ready to cut down the careless innocent who might take off his helmet to bask in the springtime sun. That's why I decided to write this diary as quickly as possible, keeping a sharp eye out to avoid being taken by surprise. I opened up my schoolboy's notebook on my bony lap to drive away fear, and every providential lull in the fighting offers me a chance to escape the present by dreaming of a postwar life or remembering our prewar days.

We succumb easily to the myth of the Golden Age. The prewar life we often found monotonous becomes in retrospect a period of unalloyed prosperity and happiness. One misses not just the sexual escapades, the free and easy ways, but the quiet evenings as well, the romantic moments, the walks along a beach—relaxed, a trifle bored, vaguely on the lookout for some excitement but without a care in the world beyond the normal concerns of an ordinary life. Like a sword of Damocles hanging over all our heads, AIDS cuts us off from both the present and the future. The constant threat of surprise bombing raids drains enjoyment from those pleasures still within our reach. It's unthinkable to dream of ever returning to those blessed, golden days, and impossible to imagine that some people back on the home front may perhaps go on enjoying life the same way we did, as if nothing at all has happened. That's why a certain bitterness may sometimes show in what I write. Unjustly, irrationally, I feel that the party's still going strong elsewhere while I'm sitting here shaking with fever. The Vietcong used to tell themselves, as they slogged through the mud, that in Saigon many of those for whom they were supposedly fighting were enjoying the good life, living off the Americans, while the women they wanted for themselves were eagerly pursuing foreigners and their collaborationists. My diehard mentality goes hand in hand with a certain puritanism—recent, in my case—that rankles in those who suffer from a kind of Cinderella complex, the feeling that everyone has gone off and left them behind to do the dirty work. My Prince Charming would be a return to health, but I'm well aware that when this is over, nothing will bring back the dead, or the carefree innocence we once knew.

When AIDS has been beaten, other sexually transmitted diseases will take its place—one of them has already been identified in Zaire—and we can't even begin to imagine their destructive potential. That's why I'm not expecting too much from the defeat of AIDS. The general relief won't last very long, and neither will the inevitable subsequent relaxation of moral standards. A new Cold War era will begin: a climate of permanent suspicion toward sexual liberty will set in, and I along with many other survivors will remain traumatized by this experience, which has taught me never to trust in nature or my own strength. It's discouraging to realize that I can never return to the infancy of my sexuality and that all the safeguards I now adopt will remain necessary precautions, even after our eventual victory. I'll never be completely demobbed; behind the Nazis, as Churchill said, are Stalin and his Cossacks.

Victory or defeat is as hard to envision as recovery or death. We find the image of decay in the physical or social body repulsive, and shrink from the grief of those left widowed, the mourning of orphaned friends. Whenever war is declared, the humiliation of defeat is never officially considered, unless it be to rally flagging spirits at a particularly critical moment in the fighting. Soldiers will die believing in the ultimate triumph of their cause, regretting only that they will never live to see the day of victory. Dying in the war against AIDS, however, contributes nothing to the enemy's defeat, unless one has participated in the experimental testing of new drugs.

People with AIDS ask each other a naïve question, one that helps us, perhaps, to carry on: When AIDS has been wiped out, what is the first thing you'll do if you get "through" it? I don't know what to answer. I'm trapped in the mental universe of the disease. AIDS has become second nature to me.

A few people will think of nothing but pleasure. Human nature will come into its own again, claiming the lifting of taboos as a reward for sufferings endured. Most of us, though, will doubtless be saved by our definitive loss of innocence when the epidemic began. Sexual Prohibition was declared during the AIDS war, and few of us count on returning to a life of "debauchery" in the event of a collective recovery. No one is naïve enough to think we're talking about the "war to end all wars." There'll always be another virus. A new generation has grown up with AIDS, like those who spent their adolescence in the shadow of both world wars. This epidemic, which has already been raging for at least seven years, holds the entire Western world hostage. We dance to its tune, and our lives are scarred by its indelible mark. Our society's youth are so traumatized that they'll never behave as we once did, never experience our former outlook on sex and life.

Will a deep bond have formed among the survivors? I doubt it, because the fabled solidarity of veteran soldiers is a short-lived thing, since each man becomes a separate individual again with the return of peace. Perhaps we'll remarry, take up new projects, and bit by bit our ties with other survivors will be broken. The day will come when we won't recognize our onetime hospital roommate out of AIDS uniform, when he brings us our brunch in a restaurant where he's back waiting on tables. The famous dancer will drive by in a limo with his new postwar friends, without seeing the former comrade with whom he once chatted familiarly in their doctor's waiting room. We won't talk about those who never came back, at first out of discretion, then from fear of boring our listeners, and finally through sheer indifference. Of course, we'll still lay flowers on the tombs of soldiers cut down in the bloom of youth, dressed to kill, marked as tempting and easy prey by the bright colors of their party clothes. We'll gather once a year at most before the flame of the Unknown AIDS Patient. It took the American authorities ten years to build a monument to their soldiers killed in Vietnam. I doubt that public opinion will demand the dedication of a statue commemorating those who died of AIDS.

The virus has dealt me a chaotic hand of cards in my life, and sometimes I have the impression that

I'm trying to turn this new deal to my advantage by attempting a ploy that would never have occurred to me before I became ill. I'm waging my personal war in the midst of a universal conflict, pursuing my crazy dream of a safe harbor when my ship's rigging is savagely buffeted by the fierce winds of AIDS. Perhaps the illness has made my mind wander; perhaps this feeling of peace I experience is only a feverish mirage, one last illusion before my system breaks down completely. I've seen too many friends and companions start out believing that their macrobiotic diets, their doses of drugs, vitamins, and medication, their carefully calculated psychological defenses had finally put them on the road to health, only to be crushed by the realization that their cancer, in remission for a year, had suddenly returned to the fray and in two weeks retaken all the ground so patiently recovered, or so they had thought, forever. That's where the enemy lies in wait for you, in that instant of despair when you're tempted to give up on all your health precautions, many of which, it's true, have much in common with the simple, age-old magic people turn to when they're suddenly confronted by a deadly menace.

Because it's certainly magical that my condition has remained stable since I began keeping this diary. Writing, even more than my psychotherapy, has helped me to understand the complexity of feeling this situation arouses in me. I'm profoundly satisfied at having ceded not a single inch of physiological ground and of having stripped a few gears in the infernal AIDS machine. What I feel is more than vain and ephemeral pride, since a new attack could instantly upset everything; it's a beneficial inner serenity. During these periods of calm, I'm at peace with the universe because I know that I might have died a thousand times over. Aside from the obvious considerations of medical logistics and mental attitude, chance has certainly played its part: I'm still alive because I've also—and above all—been lucky. All the same, I love life so much now, that life I almost lost, and I've become happier since learning to rise above material concerns. The ups and downs of my life can't be ignored, but I'm grateful to nature for the reprieve she granted me, and for a brief, blessed interlude, I'm able to look on humanity with a not too cynical eye. In such moments of grace, I might even pardon the pharisees who turn away from those already laid low, when they're not actually flailing at them with their crooks, good shepherds that they are.

From now on I prefer to channel this new energy toward those for whom this book is intended. It would be ridiculous to pretend that I'm writing for readers beyond the grave, like the director of *All Quiet on the Western Front*, who superimposes a parade of fallen heroes across the screen at the end of the film. Am I then writing for the living, my

brothers-in-arms? They'd surely have much more to
say, especially those who have suffered worse trials
than I and looked death even closer in the face. They
might reproach me for presenting such a banal, innocuous, one might almost say idyllic picture of a
disease that has ravaged them so viciously. We each
have a different perspective on our battlefield and
the war as a whole. Many might object, if they ever
read this book, that it lacks depth, that I talk more
about myself than about the cause of people with
AIDS, their daily humiliations and tragedies. Con-
scientious objectors will criticize the way I've mili-
tarized the conflict, and blame my latent neofascism.
Still others will claim their right to deny that courage
has any value, especially if draped in the militaristic
mantle I've chosen to don.

The main priority behind my nationalism—as
with all nationalisms—is to preserve my indepen-
dence: the sovereignty and integrity of my territory.
This is an instinctive reaction, not something arrived
at after long intellectual argument, and it has swept
away all the vacillations and uncertainties of the time
when I was still healthy and enjoyed the pleasures
of life. Sometimes, in these pages, I feel like a
prophet preaching a humanitarian messianism, eager to help those who suffer from the same malady
to follow my example and free themselves from the
double tyranny of AIDS and society. It wouldn't
take much to make me think I'd received a mission

from on high to awaken their downtrodden patriotism, rousing them like Joan of Arc from their unconscious pessimism. This impetus is born of the pain and distress suffered after a cataclysm, a defeat. We ought to take our revenge, because if we allow ourselves to lose we'll be the last homosexuals, which is what our enemies are hoping for, more or less explicitly. Sometimes I see myself as a doctrinarian intoxicated by his own grand principles and convinced that those unmoved by his injunctions are rushing headlong to their ruin. I, the proud possessor of the secret of survival—I'd look like an idiot once back among the dying!

I do not have a martyr's vocation, unless we're talking about those who go down fighting. A taste for the excitement only danger can provide is a characteristic of narcissism, my therapist tells me. To hell with modesty! A hero by definition must speak and make known his valorous deeds. Have I really been keeping this diary so that I can preen and strike poses? An autohagiography?

But then, haven't I written this book with still another "reader" in mind? In fact, I've written a paean to my illness. I address AIDS itself, I challenge it as fiercely as I can, in a voice that trembles ever so slightly, to prove that I won't go quietly, that I'll fight back, even if I'm half in love with my tormentor and captivated by the heat of battle. I thought I'd seen everything, and then I realized that civilian life had not prepared me for hand-to-hand combat with death. If I write to AIDS, it's in the hope that the virus will read my words, understand them, and spare me. A clumsy invocation to the God of War, a prayer like those composed by soldiers' mothers, who take care not to reproach Mars for allowing the carnage to begin, begging only that he spare one single life, that of their son, even at the cost of all the others. I'm trying my hand at a similar stratagem, attempting to convince my jailer that I can make him live on, "such virtue hath my pen," even after the discovery of the drugs that will seal his fate and which alone can sunder the accursed couple we've become. There must be love between us, because there once was jealousy. I was jealous of Oliver's AIDS: it was more spectacular than mine. It was no longer Oliver whom I desired, but his AIDS. This long love letter to AIDS is both a weapon and a white flag that I wave to indicate a desire to parley— but not to surrender. Bearing witness to my terror and that of an entire generation, this diary is also the expression of our will to mastery. The laurel crowns I weave ostensibly for AIDS have a secret purpose: to strangle and annihilate it, to make it vomit up its prey, to break its hold on my neck all stained with purplish-black lesions. We've got a death grip on each other's throat, since the ritual act of writing gives me, like David's slingshot, an unexpected advantage over this seemingly omnipotent adversary.

Even if I do wind up dying of AIDS, like all the others, I'm no longer afraid of it, because these pages have purified me, given meaning—at least for me—to these last three years of care, grief, and mourning, a meaning that is intensely personal. I shall have died for a cause, faithful to the last: the acceptance of my strengths and weaknesses, my respect for my own homosexuality and that of others, the celebration of my personality, of the choices I've made, of my love for myself and, through myself, for all humanity. (A piece of bravura kitsch that every patriotic speech must include as part of its conclusion.)

I stepped outside reality when I entered the world of AIDS, which created a feeling of displacement favorable to action as well as reflection. I won't be the first to fall in love with war. That's the limit, I've really gone crazy; I've stepped so far out of line that I've switched sides and gone over to the enemy camp. I tell myself that I'm trying to use the very strength of the epidemic for my own ends. The truth is that what I once thought I loved, what gave me pleasure, has turned out to be less fascinating and attractive than this new wartime reality. My chastity is that of a macho warrior who finds the company of women rather drab compared with the violent and varied pleasures of action. No relationship can

ever be as thrilling as my bond with AIDS. The god
Pan may inspire panic, but he is also a great sexual
principle, and the source of the martial frenzy that
possesses me. I was captivated by this madness even
before it broke out, like a country drawn helplessly
into war, hypnotized by the horror of the catastro-
phe that lies ahead. And finally, even less gloriously,
I think that my illness can be comfortable. I live in
AIDS the way a hermit crab uses a shell to protect
its soft, defenseless body. Curled up inside the folds
of the AIDS carapace, I have used these fragile scraps
of thought, gathered day after day, to block up the
entrance to my shell.

Within my life, the parenthetical digression of
disease has opened wide its jaws. This illness offers
us an abridged version of existence that is also a
bitter parody. Our new date of birth is the day when
we discovered that we carried AIDS inside us. We
know that, from then on, hours count as days, and
months as years. Our return to childhood is a hand-
icap this time around, because at first we have no
idea how to channel our energies; but if we can
survive the first few months, our innate strength will
reassert itself. The danger is all the greater when the
patient fighting back is inexperienced and unreal-
istic. A year ago I was still complaining about having
lapsed prematurely into the rhythm of retirement,
but since then I've learned to appreciate this slower
pace, making allowances for simple trepidation as

well as profoundly felt moments of life itself. The proximity of danger is the beginning of wisdom, and my renunciation is not only spontaneous but also, at present, desired. Even if our death comes early on, we will have lived all the ages of man. The corpse of a youth of twenty-five, exhausted by dehydration, bears a strange resemblance to that of a disfigured old man. Our remains are ageless.

The acceleration of the aging process is inherent in every crisis. The failure of the immune system in AIDS patients has often been compared to its breakdown in the elderly, whose abilities to resist disease dwindle rapidly, setting them on an ever-quickening course toward death. AIDS ages, and it does so absolutely. Body, spirit, virility: all come under attack. Like the elderly who go into a decline after their retirement, people with AIDS are tempted to give up making plans and simply bury themselves alive in the ruins. I've aged ten years in the last twelve months, and the dark circles under my eyes might make it seem, despite my reclusive existence, that I'm running riot in debauchery, unless, of course, this sudden change is something like the one that overtook Dorian Gray. The faces of people with AIDS are as many secret portraits revealed by their illness, pictures that the braver ones among us dare approach and contemplate. In our morbidly guilty frame of mind, each viral torment seems to correspond to a superfluous coupling from the past. An attack of diarrhea for the Californian surfer, a bad cough for the barman in his leather outfit, a raging temperature for the Puerto Rican out on the piers. In war novels, beardless adolescents return from the front with the self-assurance, the careworn faces, and the existential lassitude of those who have had to live beyond their strength for a long time. Their souls are scarred, but resolute. In the same way, I've seen young AIDS patients show a maturity well beyond their years, a sense of values it takes some people an entire lifetime to acquire.

I'm reading an English book entitled *AIDS Survival*. The author's tone is both courageous and detached, and it reminds me of the resilience of Londoners under the Blitz. I now know that English AIDS patients must suffer not only assaults from the virus but also the attacks of Fleet Street, those tabloids that go after the victims instead of the epidemic. The shame of English AIDS victims was brought home to me not long ago when I saw on television that no patient had been willing to be filmed with Princess Diana at the inauguration of the first hospital wing devoted to the treatment of AIDS in England. The frustrated cameras could show nothing but beds empty of their intended occupants and the princess surrounded by officials in the pink of health. How heavily English homophobia must weigh on those AIDS victims, whom I see as gallant fighter pilots in the RAF, to make them hide their faces when a future queen of England comes to shake their hands! Who is the Churchill who will give us the courage to shake off the hordes of Lilliputians who torment us with their small minds and even smaller hearts?

Beyond my first patriotic horizon—my own survival—I see another Jerusalem for which many are still fighting unawares: the Cities of Salt, where we have found so many pleasures, and so much comfort in a hostile world. This second native country is our homosexual tribe (as one might say, the tribe of Judah), and we belong to it from childhood, an affiliation that seems as natural to us as our own bodies, even though those who are outside this bond see it as strange, comical, or repulsive. Like those young Jews who return to the roots of Hebraic tradition, I'm tempted to rekindle the guttering flame of homosexuality. How can we recover, in the midst of this epidemic, the pride and dignity of fifteen or twenty years ago? The people of Israel have suffered appalling calamities throughout history, and miraculously they have endured. It seems to me that homosexuals in the West should show the same courage and tenacity against our own Nebuchadnezzar, AIDS, and stop seeing homosexuality as the cause of their current plight. We must cure ourselves, not by turning away from the poisoned well of homosexuality, but by drawing from it new reserves of spiritual strength, merely filtering out the dangers inherent in careless sexual activity.

We should not allow the virus to dismember our homeland, the sense of community that has been so precious to us in our past trials. Surrounded by hostility, like Israel since biblical times, we should show a united front and take advantage of our common bonds. Since the beginning of this diary, I've thus been speaking, consciously or not, as a nationalist of homosexuality. After all, despite the extreme diversity of the gay community, I almost always feel an affinity with my fellow citizens wherever I go, the way a Frenchman or an American shares a common background with any compatriot encountered abroad. There are so many things we don't have to explain, justify, or defend among ourselves. It's this consensus within the gay community that should provide the basis for our counterattack against those who eagerly seek to exploit our fears and uncertainties. Day after day, we must burn our Trojan horse to ashes and in its place construct the Ark of our Covenant. The war memorial to those felled by AIDS should logically resemble the Wailing Wall, where true believers pray in memory of ordeals visited upon their people by God. Like Job, we should refuse to curse our fate, instead devoting all our strength to surviving until both God and the devil tire of tormenting us and the virus is expelled from our desecrated Temple.

MY BODY, MY BEIRUT

WITHIN EACH ORGAN of my body, viruses and
toxic drugs have been like armies locked in fratricidal
combat for more than three years now. All these
cells, and even the viruses, the amoebas, parasites,
mycoses, blemishes, they're all a part of me; I am
made of them, and this intestinal strife is played out
in my digestive tract. For a long time I was just a
passive spectator at these gun battles raging up and
down my streets. Many people with AIDS are content to learn what's going on in their own veins by
watching TV news reports, leaving their fate to be
decided by the various factions in a vast army of
doctors and health-care workers. Of course, my sym-
pathies lie with the forces of life, but I rely on specialists to restore order in my state. Like many
Lebanese, who provide a fascinated captive audience
for the apocalyptic struggle between the different
denominational groups that prevent their society
from functioning, thereby robbing their countrymen of work and pleasure, I find it difficult to feel
personally involved in this scattershot battle that yet
manages to completely upset my existence. All I can
say is that I've chosen my side by instinct, and I'm
staying put, just as stubbornly as the citizens of Bei-

rut. I'm quite willing to camp out amid the ruins, piecing together a semblance of normal life, going to work with stomach cramps, going out for the evening with friends (after taking enough pills to choke a horse), at the mercy of an attack of diarrhea or a sudden feeling of exhaustion, like the Lebanese who risk being stopped at an intersection at any moment by militiamen armed with machine guns and ready to turn a pleasant outing into a nightmare. Now I can understand those civilians who used to confound me by their seemingly irrational persistence in clinging to a phantom city clearly in the throes of disintegration. If they left, they'd feel as though they were deserting a beloved country. I know what those people are going through, I know how they feel, and I know that their obstinacy has no more to do with logic than has my own insistence on pretending that everything is as normal as possible, when even eighteen months ago I would have found my present existence surreal and absolutely unlivable. In memory of the happiness my life and body afforded me before this war broke out, I feel an almost visceral obligation to settle in for a long siege, for as long as it takes.

I can accept this situation all the more readily because the deterioration of my body and my living conditions has been a slow, gradual process, as it has been for Beirut, so that my daily sacrifices are quite tolerable. It's only when I look back over a longer period of time that I see how the accumulation of these trials has devastated my personal topography, redrawing the map of my city along such unfamiliar lines. In this urban guerrilla war, the ranks of fighters may be suddenly thinned; a viral sniper lying in ambush on a roof can pick off healthy carriers in a flash, men who thought themselves in good shape and safe from stray bullets.

Obviously, this decrepit body now bears only a faint resemblance to the harmonious proportions of the past. Like the very aged, the veterans of AIDS retain traces of their youthful beauty, evoking graceful cities not yet completely disfigured in a senseless war. If I ever come to resemble Berlin in May 1945, it will perhaps be time for me to poison us both, AIDS and me, in our bunker.

New York, July 14, 1987

Acknowledgments

Since this book was a medico-literary undertaking, I am grateful both to those who take care of me, thanks to whom I have had the time and energy to write, and to those who have surrounded me with their redoubled affection, encouraging me in my decision to write this diary. Let me mention first those who have believed in my chances for survival: my doctors, Joseph Sonnabend and Donald Kotler; Daniel Altilio and Helen Ferlazzo, the visiting nurses who have been tending to me twice a week for two years now; my ophthalmologist, Steven Teich, and my psychoanalyst, Natalie Becker, who was instrumental in my decision to write this book. I have not forgotten what Dr. Duflo and the medical team headed by Dr. Gentilini accomplished in France two years ago in the way of retarding the progress of my illness.

The moral support of those close to me, whom I have dragged into action on my private battlefield, has been just as precious to me. Kristine Dreuilhe, of course, but also Jean-Michel Sivry, Reine Locci, and Veronica Selver, who followed closely every stage in the writing of this book, which has benefited a great deal from their valuable advice.

I'm also grateful for the suggestions of Claudine Dreuilhe, Catherine Collet, Rosemary Pugliese, Stephen Harvey, Charles-Henri Flammarion, and Fauvette van der Schoot. I was quite touched by the patience and dedication of Marie-Josée Sellier and Monique Bourassa, who took in hand the many revisions of my manuscript. And I was surprised and pleased to have been joined in my trench by Edwy Plenel, an ally who arrived in New York out of the blue at the last minute to give expert help in the editing of this text.

It is thanks to the warm and generous support of Jack-Alain Léger that my book was published in France, while this American edition is the result of the kind and patient efforts of Susan Sontag, Richard Howard, and Steve Wasserman. My particular thanks to Linda Coverdale, who instantly found the tone and style I thought this book needed to survive in English. I should like to express my appreciation to all my friends and colleagues for not having changed in their attitude toward me after I became ill.

Finally, there are two people whose real names I cannot reveal—Oliver, and Julia, his mother—because this heroic woman has chosen to spare her family the shock she herself went through. Without them, without what they taught me, I would never have learned how to pass from anger to compassion, from revolt to serenity. Thanks to them, I've understood the need to transcend sorrow and self-pity.

A Note about the Author

*Emmanuel Dreuilhe was born in Cairo in
1949 and spent his childhood in French
Indochina. He works as a translator
and lives in New York City.*